Gastroenterology
on the move

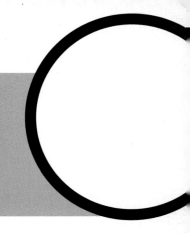

Gastroenterology
on the move

Authors: **Arash Assadsangabi,
Lucy Carroll and Andrew Irvine**
Editorial Advisor: **Keith Dear**

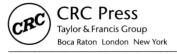

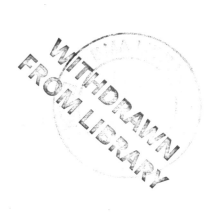

CRC Press
Taylor & Francis Group
Boca Raton London New York

CRC Press is an imprint of the
Taylor & Francis Group, an **informa** business

CRC Press
Taylor & Francis Group
6000 Broken Sound Parkway NW, Suite 300
Boca Raton, FL 33487-2742

© 2016 by Taylor & Francis Group, LLC
CRC Press is an imprint of Taylor & Francis Group, an Informa business

No claim to original U.S. Government works

Printed on acid-free paper
Version Date: 20150909

International Standard Book Number-13: 978-1-4822-5244-6 (Pack - Book and Ebook)

Visit the Taylor & Francis Web site at
http://www.taylorandfrancis.com

and the CRC Press Web site at
http://www.crcpress.com

Contents

Preface

Have you ever found gastroenterology overwhelmingly complicated? Have you struggled to recall the basics in a clinical situation? Or are you simply short of time and have exams looming? If so, this concise, practical guide will help you.

Written by doctors for doctors, this book presents information in a wide range of formats including flow charts, boxes, summary tables and colourful diagrams. No matter what your learning style is, we hope that you will find the book appealing and easy to read. We think that the innovative style will help you, the reader, to connect with this often feared topic, to learn, understand and even enjoy it, and to apply what you have learned in your clinical practice and in the pressured run-up to final examinations.

In writing the book, we have drawn on our recent personal experience as medical students and junior doctors, and hope this book will offer the less-experienced a portable and practical guide to gastroenterology that will complement larger reference texts. We hope you find it helpful!

AUTHORS

Arash Assadsangabi MD MRCP – Specialist Registrar in Gastroenterology and General Internal Medicine, Royal Hallamshire Hospital, Sheffield, UK
Lucy Carroll MBChB LLM – Foundation 1 Doctor, Huddersfield Royal Infirmary, West Yorkshire, UK
Andrew Irvine – Medical Student, University of Sheffield, Sheffield, UK

EDITORIAL ADVISOR

Keith Dear – Consultant Gastroenterologist, Chesterfield Royal Hospital, Chesterfield, UK

EDITOR-IN-CHIEF

Rory Mackinnon BSc(Hons) MBChB MRCGP – GP Partner, Dr Cloak & Partners, Southwick Health Centre, Sunderland, UK

SERIES EDITORS

Andrew MN Walker BMedSci MBChB MRCP (London) – British Heart Foundation Clinical Research Fellow and Honorary Specialist Registrar in Cardiology, University of Leeds, UK
Harriet Walker – CT1 in Plastic Surgery, Derriford Hospital, Devon, UK

Acknowledgements

We thank the editors for their invaluable help during the writing of this book, particularly Harriet Walker and Andy Walker for their contributions. Thanks also to Servier Medical Art for the use of their images for this book. We also thank Dr Andrew Hopper and Dr Rathinavel Balamurugan, who provided us several of the radiological images.

List of abbreviations

- γGT: gamma-glutamyl transferase
- ACE: antegrade colonic enema
- AFP: α-fetoprotein
- ALD: alcoholic liver disease
- ALP: alkaline phosphatase
- ALT: alanine aminotransferase
- ANA: antinuclear antibody
- APC: argon plasma coagulation
- ARDS: acute respiratory distress syndrome
- AST: aspartate aminotransferase
- AUDIT: Alcohol Use Disorders Identification Test
- AXR: abdominal X-ray
- BCLC: Barcelona Clinic Liver Cancer classification
- BMI: body mass index
- BP: blood pressure
- BSG: British Society of Gastroenterology
- CCK: cholecystokinin
- CD: Crohn's disease
- CDT: *Clostridium difficile* toxin
- CEA: carcinoembryonic antigen
- CF: cystic fibrosis
- CMV: cytomegalovirus
- CNS: central nervous system
- COPD: chronic obstructive pulmonary disease
- CRC: colorectal cancer
- CRP: C-reactive protein
- CSF: cerebrospinal fluid
- CT: computed tomography
- CXR: chest X-ray
- DEXA: dual-energy X-ray absorptiometry
- DF: discriminate function
- DRE: digital rectal examination
- EBV: Epstein–Barr virus
- ED: emergency department
- EGG: electrogastrography
- EMA: endomysial antibody
- EMR: endoscopic mucosal resection
- ERCP: endoscopic retrograde cholangiopancreatography
- ESD: endoscopic submucosal dissection

- ESR: erythrocyte sedimentation rate
- EUS: endoscopic ultrasound
- FAP: familial adenomatous polyposis
- FAST: Fast Alcohol Screening Test
- FBC: full blood count
- FOB: faecal occult blood
- FODMAP: fermentable oligo-di-monosaccharides and polyols
- FSH: follicle-stimulating hormone
- FVL: factor V Leiden
- GI: gastrointestinal
- GIST: gastrointestinal stromal tumours
- GOJ: gastro-oesophageal junction
- GORD: gastro-oesophageal reflux disease
- GP: general practitioner
- Hb: haemoglobin
- HCC: hepatocellular carcinoma
- HLA: human leukocyte antigen
- HNPCC: hereditary non-polyposis colorectal carcinoma
- HR: heart rate
- HUS: haemolytic uraemic syndrome
- IBD: inflammatory bowel disease
- IBS: irritable bowel syndrome
- IEL: intra-epithelial lymphocyte
- IgA: immunoglobulin A
- IV: intravenous
- IVC: inferior vena cava
- LDH: lactate dehydrogenase
- LFT: liver function test
- LH: luteinizing hormone
- LOS: lower oesophageal sphincter
- MALT: mucosa-associated lymphoid tissue
- MCV: mean corpuscular volume
- MC&S: microscopy, culture and sensitivity
- MELD: Model for End-Stage Liver Disease
- MMSE: Mini-Mental State Examination
- MND: motor neurone disease
- MRA: magnetic resonance angiography
- MRCP: magnetic resonance cholangiopancreatography
- MS: multiple sclerosis
- MUST: Malnutrition Universal Screening Tool
- NAAT: nucleic acid amplification test
- NAFLD: non-alcoholic fatty liver disease

- NASH: non-alcoholic steatohepatitis
- NBM: nil by mouth
- NG: nasogastric
- NJ: nasojejunal
- NSAID: non-steroidal anti-inflammatory drug
- OGD: oesophago-gastro-duodenoscopy
- PAS: periodic acid–Schiff
- PBC: primary biliary cirrhosis
- PCOS: polycystic ovary syndrome
- PCR: polymerase chain reaction
- PEG: percutaneous endoscopic gastrostomy
- PEJ: percutaneous endoscopic jejunostomy
- PICC: peripherally inserted central catheter
- Plt: platelet
- PPI: proton pump inhibitor
- PR: pulse rate
- PSC: primary sclerosing cholangitis
- PT: prothrombin time
- PTC: percutaneous transhepatic cholangiography
- PTH: parathyroid hormone
- QDS: four times per day
- RR: respiration rate
- SBP: spontaneous bacterial peritonitis
- SIBO: small intestinal bacterial overgrowth
- SLE: systemic lupus erythematosus
- SMA: smooth muscle antibody
- SRUS: solitary rectal ulcer syndrome
- SSRI: selective serotonin reuptake inhibitor
- TACE: transcatheter arterial chemo-embolization
- TB: tuberculosis
- TCA: tricyclic antidepressant
- TFT: thyroid function test
- TI: terminal ileum
- TIBC: total iron-binding capacity
- TIPS: transjugular intrahepatic portosystemic shunt
- TNM: tumour, nodes, metastases
- TPN: total parenteral nutrition
- TSH: thyroid-stimulating hormone
- tTG: tissue transglutaminase
- U&E: urea and electrolytes
- UC: ulcerative colitis
- UKELD: United Kingdom model for End-Stage Liver Disease

- UOS: upper oesophageal sphincter
- USS: ultrasound scan
- UTI: urinary tract infection
- VLDL: very-low-density lipoprotein
- WCC: white cell count

List of figures

An explanation of the text

The book is divided into two parts: one covers the clinical aspects of gastroenterology and the other is a self-assessment section. We have used bullet points to keep the text concise and supplemented this with a range of diagrams, pictures and MICRO-boxes (explained below).

Where possible we have endeavoured to include treatment options for the conditions covered. Nevertheless, drug sensitivities and clinical practices are constantly under review, so always check your local guidelines for up-to-date information.

You will find the following resources useful to learn more about the drugs mentioned in this book:

- BNF (https://www.medicinescomplete.com/about/subscribe.htm)
- eMC (http://www.medicines.org.uk/emc/)

MICRO-facts

These boxes expand on the text and contain clinically relevant facts and memorable summaries of the essential information.

MICRO-print

These boxes contain additional information to the text that may interest certain readers but is not essential for everybody to learn.

MICRO-case

These boxes contain clinical cases relevant to the text and include a number of summary bullet points to highlight the key learning objectives.

MICRO-reference

These boxes contain references to important clinical research and national guidance.

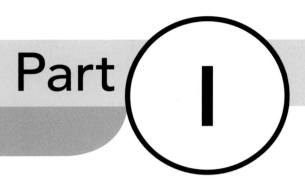

Part I

Gastroenterology

1 Common upper GI presentations

1.1 DYSPEPSIA

DEFINITION

- Commonly referred to as indigestion.
- Gives rise to characteristic symptoms:
  - Upper abdominal (epigastric) pain or burning.
  - Bloating and early satiety.
  - Nausea.
  - Heartburn.
  - Belching.

> **MICRO-reference**
> See the Rome III diagnostic criteria for further information on the classification of dyspepsia: http://www.romecriteria.org/assets/pdf/19_RomeIII_apA_885-898.pdf

CLINICAL FEATURES

- History:
  - Site of the pain:
    - Retrosternal discomfort: oesophageal spasm, gastro-oesophageal reflux disease (GORD), hiatus hernia.
    - Epigastric pain: peptic ulcer.
    - Radiating to the right shoulder: gallstones.
  - Exacerbating factors:
    - Eating: gastric ulcer, GORD.
    - Consumption of fatty foods: gallstones.
    - Lying flat: GORD.
  - Relieving factors:
    - Eating: duodenal ulcer.

- Examination:
  - Weight loss: oesophageal carcinoma, gastric carcinoma.
  - Obese/pregnant patient: increased risk of GORD, hiatus hernia.
  - Anaemia: bleeding peptic ulcer, malignancy.
  - Virchow's node: gastric carcinoma.
  - Jaundice: gallstones, malignancy.
  - Epigastric mass: gastric carcinoma.

MICRO-facts

When giving antacids, aluminium compounds may cause constipation whereas magnesium compounds have a laxative effect.
When given together, this balances out the GI side effects.

MICRO-facts

Red flags for dyspepsia:

- Weight loss (unintentional)
- Dysphagia
- Melaena
- Haematemesis
- Suspicious barium study
- Iron deficiency anaemia (IDA)
- Epigastric mass
- Persistent vomiting

Gastroenterology

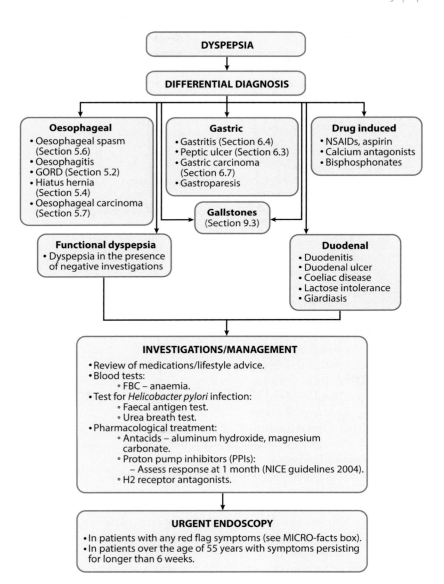

Figure 1.1 Immediate management of dyspepsia.

1.2 DYSPHAGIA

DEFINITION

- Difficulty in swallowing.

CLINICAL FEATURES

- History:
    - Onset of dysphagia:
        - Acute onset: foreign body, oesophageal spasm.
        - Intermittent: oesophageal spasm.
        - Chronic progressive: oesophageal stricture, oesophageal carcinoma, mediastinal/lung tumours, motor neurone disease (MND), systemic sclerosis.
    - Nature of the food:
        - Solids and liquids from presentation:
            - More likely to be due to mechanical failure: achalasia, myasthenia gravis.
        - Solids progressing to include liquids:
            - Usually due to a progressive process (see causes of chronic dysphagia).
    - Stage at which dysphagia occurs during swallowing:
        - Difficulty in initiating a swallow:
            - Disorders of the pharynx or mouth: oral carcinoma, neurological causes.
        - After a few seconds:
            - Oesophageal causes: achalasia, oesophagitis.
    - Associated symptoms:
        - Odynophagia (pain on swallowing): oesophagitis.
        - Weight loss:
            - May be due to inadequate intake of food due to dysphagia.
            - May be caused by pharyngeal carcinoma, oesophageal carcinoma, extrinsic compression from carcinoma of the lung or thyroid goitre.
        - Vomiting/regurgitation: pharyngeal pouch, reflux oesophagitis/ hiatus hernia, achalasia.
    - Associated medical conditions (e.g. MND, MS, thyroid disease etc.).
    - Previous surgery (e.g. oesophagectomy).
- Examination:
    - Signs of malnutrition/weight loss: malignancy, MND (muscle wasting).
    - Inspection of the mouth: oral carcinoma, candidiasis.

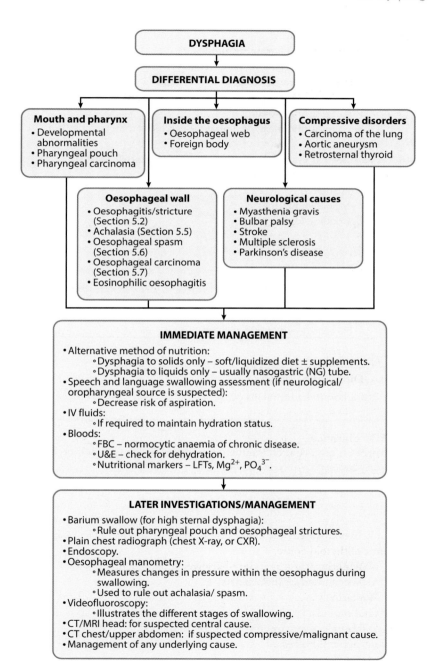

Figure 1.2 Immediate management of dysphagia.

- Hoarseness of voice:
  - May indicate a laryngeal problem.
  - Carcinoma of the lung compressing the recurrent laryngeal nerve.
- Observation of swallowing:
  - Pain on swallowing.
  - Regurgitation/choking.
- Upper abdominal mass: oesophageal carcinoma, metastatic liver deposits.
- Neurological signs: fatigue, tongue wasting, muscle wasting.
- Features of systemic illness:
  - Anaemia.
  - Lymphadenopathy.
  - Systemic sclerosis.

COMPLICATIONS

- Malnutrition.
- Dehydration.

1.3 UPPER GI BLEEDING

EPIDEMIOLOGY

- Incidence is 84–172 per 100,000 per year.
- 50–70,000 hospital admissions per year.

MICRO-reference

See the NICE guideline on the management of upper GI bleeding here: http://guidance.nice.org.uk/CG141

RISK FACTORS

- Chronic liver disease.
- Medications:
  - NSAIDs.
  - Aspirin and other antiplatelets.
  - Warfarin.
  - Oral steroids.
  - SSRIs (selective serotonin reuptake inhibitors).
- Previous upper GI bleed.
- Upper GI malignancy.
- *Helicobacter pylori* infection: increased peptic ulcer risk.

CLINICAL FEATURES

- Haematemesis: vomiting of fresh blood.
- Melaena: altered blood passed per rectum.
- Symptoms of shock (if severe):
  - Increased heart rate.
  - Low blood pressure.
  - Cold, clammy skin.
  - Increased respiratory rate.

MICRO-print
The Blatchford Score (see table) is recommended by NICE for risk assessment of upper GI bleed patients at first assessment. A score of 0 is considered low risk. Scores of 1 or more are considered higher risk. The higher the score, the greater the chance of intervention being required. A score of 6 is associated with a 50% chance that intervention will be required.

BLATCHFORD SCORE VARIABLES		SCORE
Urea	≥6.5 to <8.0	2
	≥8.0 to <10.0	3
	≥10.0 to ≤25.0	4
	>25.0	6
Haemoglobin (men)	≥12.0 to <13.0	1
	≥10.0 to <12.0	3
	<10.0	6
Haemoglobin (women)	≥10.0 to <12.0	1
	<10.0	6
Systolic blood pressure (mmHg)	100–109	1
	90–99	2
	<90	3
Other markers	Pulse ≥100 (per min)	1
	Presentation with melaena	1
	Presentation with syncope	2
	Hepatic disease	2
	Cardiac failure	2

continued...

Gastroenterology

continued...

The Rockall Score contains both pre-endoscopic and post-endoscopic variables and is used to predict mortality and risk of rebleeding and is recommended for post-endoscopic risk management by NICE.

MANAGEMENT

- Initial management (see Figure 1.3):
  - Risk assessment is important:
    - Blatchford Score – recommended for pre-endoscopy risk assessment by NICE (see MICRO-print box).
    - Rockall Score – recommended by NICE for post-endoscopy risk assessment (see MICRO-print box).
- Endoscopic management:
  - Identify the source of bleeding: not always identified.
  - Treatment:
    - Mechanical: clips.
    - Thermal: heater probe, argon plasma coagulation (APC).
    - Injection therapy: adrenaline, thrombin.
    - Variceal treatment: banding/injection of cyanoacrylate glue.
- Radiological management:
  - Embolization of artery in non-variceal bleeds:
    - Indicated if endoscopic management is unsuccessful.
  - Transjugular intrahepatic portosystemic shunt (TIPS) (see Chapter 4):
    - Indicated in refractory variceal bleeding.
- Surgical management:
  - Only around 2% of patients require surgery.
  - Indications:
    - Recurrent bleeds.
    - High-risk lesions (posterior duodenal ulcers).
    - Multiple/large ulcers.
    - Uncontrollable bleeding.
  - Surgical management is associated with a high mortality (around 30%).
- Other treatments:
  - Balloon tamponade of varices (e.g. Minnesota tube):
    - Used if bleeding continues despite banding.
    - Gastric and oesophageal balloons are inflated to compress varices and stop acute bleeding.
    - Often used as a temporary measure prior to TIPS.

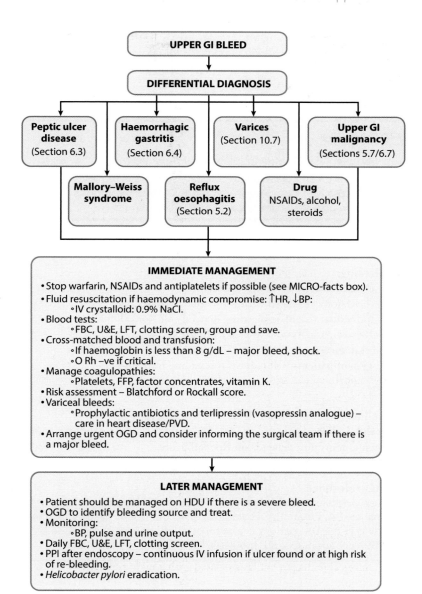

Figure 1.3 Immediate management of upper GI bleeding.

- Oesophageal stenting for varices:
  - Alternative to balloon tamponade for refractory bleeding.
  - A covered, removable oesophageal stent is inserted to compress oesophageal varices.
  - Removed 6–8 weeks later.

MICRO-facts

Stop warfarin, NSAIDs and antiplatelets if possible:

- If patient is on anti platelets for coronary stenting in the last 12 months, then discuss with cardiologist – high rate of stent thrombosis.
- Low-dose aspirin can be restarted once bleeding is controlled.

COMPLICATIONS

- Re-bleeding:
  - Overall around 13% will re-bleed:
    - Majority re-bleed within the first 72 hours.
  - Individual risk of re-bleeding depends on Rockall Score.
  - 40% of patients who re-bleed will die.
- Blood transfusion:
  - 43% of patients will require at least one transfusion.

PROGNOSIS

- Overall mortality is around 10%.
- Mortality is 26% if the patient is an inpatient and 7% in new admissions.
- Individual mortality depends on Rockall Score.

MICRO-reference

Data on complications and mortality in upper GI bleeding taken from: Hearnshaw SA, Logan RA, Lowe D, et al. Acute upper gastrointestinal bleeding in the UK: patient characteristics, diagnoses and outcomes in the 2007 UK audit. *Gut* 2011; 60(10): 1327–1335.

1.4 VOMITING

PATHOPHYSIOLOGY

- Initiation of vomiting:
  - The vomiting centre is located in the lateral reticular formation of the medulla on the floor of the fourth ventricle of the brain.

- Vomiting is mediated by the GI system:
  - Impulses from the pharynx, stomach and small bowel are relayed to the vomiting centre via the vagus and sympathetic nerves.
  - When activated, the vomiting centre relays impulses to higher cortical centres to provoke the sensation of nausea:
    - ○ Efferent impulses to the stomach inhibit antral and small bowel contractions, promote diaphragmatic and intercostal muscle contractions and close the glottis causing retching.
    - ○ Vomiting occurs when forceful retrograde peristalsis of the jejunum pushes enteric contents into the stomach, followed by relaxation of the LOS, resulting in propulsion of the gastric contents into the mouth.

MICRO-facts

- The enteric nervous system controls the GI tract under influence from the central nervous system (via autonomic nerves) and hormones.
- It is composed of two nerve plexuses: the submucosal (Meissner's) plexus and the myenteric (Auerbach's) plexus.
- The enteric nervous system has both sensory and motor components, allowing it to monitor the luminal environment and alter GI secretions and motility accordingly.

MICRO-print
Physiology of vomiting:

- Parasympathetic output – increased salivation in order to protect tooth enamel from acidic stomach contents.
- Sympathetic output – increased heart rate and sweating.
- Motor output – responsible for the physical act of vomiting.
- Neurotransmitters – histamine, dopamine, serotonin, neurokinin, vasopressin.

DIFFERENTIAL DIAGNOSIS

- Important to remember both GI and non-GI causes (see Figure 1.4).
- Wide differential covering many systems (systems review is essential).

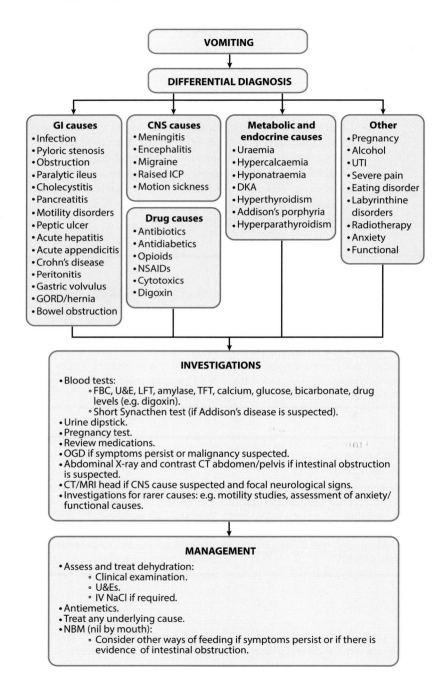

VOMITING

DIFFERENTIAL DIAGNOSIS

GI causes
- Infection
- Pyloric stenosis
- Obstruction
- Paralytic ileus
- Cholecystitis
- Pancreatitis
- Motility disorders
- Peptic ulcer
- Acute hepatitis
- Acute appendicitis
- Crohn's disease
- Peritonitis
- Gastric volvulus
- GORD/hernia
- Bowel obstruction

CNS causes
- Meningitis
- Encephalitis
- Migraine
- Raised ICP
- Motion sickness

Drug causes
- Antibiotics
- Antidiabetics
- Opioids
- NSAIDs
- Cytotoxics
- Digoxin

Metabolic and endocrine causes
- Uraemia
- Hypercalcaemia
- Hyponatraemia
- DKA
- Hyperthyroidism
- Addison's porphyria
- Hyperparathyroidism

Other
- Pregnancy
- Alcohol
- UTI
- Severe pain
- Eating disorder
- Labyrinthine disorders
- Radiotherapy
- Anxiety
- Functional

INVESTIGATIONS
- Blood tests:
  - FBC, U&E, LFT, amylase, TFT, calcium, glucose, bicarbonate, drug levels (e.g. digoxin).
  - Short Synacthen test (if Addison's disease is suspected).
- Urine dipstick.
- Pregnancy test.
- Review medications.
- OGD if symptoms persist or malignancy suspected.
- Abdominal X-ray and contrast CT abdomen/pelvis if intestinal obstruction is suspected.
- CT/MRI head if CNS cause suspected and focal neurological signs.
- Investigations for rarer causes: e.g. motility studies, assessment of anxiety/ functional causes.

MANAGEMENT
- Assess and treat dehydration:
  - Clinical examination.
  - U&Es.
  - IV NaCl if required.
- Antiemetics.
- Treat any underlying cause.
- NBM (nil by mouth):
  - Consider other ways of feeding if symptoms persist or if there is evidence of intestinal obstruction.

Figure 1.4 Immediate management of vomiting.

Gastroenterology

CLINICAL FEATURES

- History:
  - Vomiting:
    - Timing:
      - Early morning in a female: pregnancy.
      - Post chemotherapy/surgery.
    - Relationship to meals:
      - Soon after: achalasia or other oesophageal causes, pharyngeal pouch, pancreatitis or cholecystitis.
      - Delayed: gastroparesis, gastric outflow obstruction, distal obstruction.
    - Amount.
    - Content:
      - Coffee grounds: dark brown vomit, similar in appearance to coffee grounds, which is a result of blood coming into contact with gastric acid.
      - Undigested food: achalasia.
      - Partially digested food: gastric outflow obstruction, gastroparesis.
      - Bilious: obstruction distal to sphincter of Oddi.
      - Blood stained: mucosal damage.
  - Associated symptoms:
    - Pain: ulcers, obstruction, pancreatitis, cholecystitis.
    - Weight loss: malignancy, eating disorder.
    - Diarrhoea: infection.
    - Headaches, visual disturbance, neck stiffness: CNS cause.
    - Tinnitus and vertigo: inner ear cause.
- Examination:
  - Tinkling bowel sounds: obstruction.
  - Succussion splash: gastric outlet obstruction.
  - Abdominal mass: malignancy.
  - Tenderness: infection or inflammation.
  - Distension: obstruction.
  - Fever: infection or inflammation.
  - Jaundice: cholecystitis.
  - Neurological signs: CNS cause.

COMPLICATIONS

- Severe dehydration.
- Electrolyte imbalances:
  - Hypochloraemic alkalosis with hypokalaemia.

- Mallory–Weiss tears.
- Oesophagitis.
- Oesophageal rupture.

MICRO-facts

Concerning features of vomiting:
- Blood-stained vomit
- Bile-stained vomit
- Weight loss
- Tinkling bowel sounds
- Neurological signs

MICRO-facts

Classes of anti emetics:
- Dopamine antagonists: domperidone, metoclopramide
- Histamine antagonists: cyclizine
- Antiserotonergics: ondansetron
- Antimuscarinics: hyoscine
- Cannabinoids: nabilone

MICRO-case

A 42-year-old unemployed man was found by his wife lying in bed surrounded by blood-stained vomit. He was easily rousable although this triggered further vomiting, this time with large amounts of fresh blood. An ambulance was called and the patient was admitted through the ED.

A thorough history was taken and he denied any abdominal pain. He remembers feeling unwell and began vomiting, but his memory of further events is poor. His stool has been normal and he denies taking any NSAIDs or aspirin. He has no history of reflux symptoms.

On further questioning, he admits to drinking alcohol every day for the last 4 years since being made redundant. He says he drinks around 1 pint of strong cider a day, but his wife interjects and says it is actually 2 litres of strong cider. He has never been diagnosed with liver problems.

On examination, he appears slightly pale. His blood pressure is 95/75 mmHg, pulse 105 bpm, respiratory rate 18 breaths per minute. He is noted to have palmar erythema, several spider naevi and slight gynaecomastia.

continued...

continued...

He is stabilized in the ED with 1 litre of 0.9% sodium chloride, which returns his blood pressure and heart rate to normal limits. Bloods are taken for FBC, U&E, LFT, clotting screen and group and save. It is felt the bleeding may be due to varices, so terlipressin is started in an attempt to reduce portal pressure. Prophylactic antibiotics are given to reduce risk of subsequent infection.

The patient's FBC shows an Hb of 8 g/dL and a platelet count of 45. His LFTs give a bilirubin of 30 μmol/L, albumin 30 g/L, ALT 65 IU/L and γGT of 452 IU/L. Prothrombin time is increased by 6 seconds. He is given a platelet transfusion, fresh frozen plasma and vitamin K.

On the basis of the blood results, the Blatchford Score is calculated to be 11 and the case is discussed with the on-call gastroenterology team. It is decided to take the patient to endoscopy to confirm and treat the cause of the bleed. He is found to have large varices that are banded to prevent further bleeding. OGD also shows portal hypertensive gastropathy (a characteristic set of mucosal changes seen in patients with portal hypertension).

After the endoscopy, the patient is transferred to the high dependency unit, where he is started on a number of new medications. Pabrinex is given IV for 3 days to replace B vitamins and reduce the risk of developing Wernicke's encephalopathy. To prevent symptoms of alcohol withdrawal, he is also started on a reducing regime of chlordiazepoxide.

Key points:

- Upper GI bleeding can be the first presentation of alcoholic liver disease. Although many patients with variceal bleeds will be known to have liver disease, a proportion will not.
- Stabilization of patients presenting with upper GI bleeds is important pre-endoscopy. Endoscopy puts stress on the cardiovascular and respiratory systems, so ideally patients need to be in the best condition possible before the procedure is carried out. Unfortunately this is not always possible and stopping bleeding may take priority in certain situations.
- Risk assessment is important. Using the Blatchford Score predicts the need for intervention and so is useful in formulating management plans.
- Other causes of liver disease should be considered in such cases. There is an increased risk of several liver conditions among heavy drinkers (see Chapter 10).
- Care of patients post-endoscopy is important. Recognizing and treating symptoms of Wernicke's and alcohol withdrawal prevents increased morbidity and mortality.

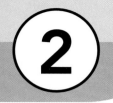

Common small bowel presentations

2.1 MALABSORPTION

DEFINITION

- Inability of the small intestine to absorb nutrients passing through it secondary to a wide range of pathologies.

PATHOPHYSIOLOGY

- Physiology of normal absorption:
    - Functions of the small bowel are digestion and absorption of carbohydrates, fats and proteins together with the absorption of vitamins, minerals, electrolytes and water.
    - Duodenal enterocytes release bicarbonate to neutralize stomach acid, increasing the pH to an optimum level for enzyme function.
    - Pancreatic enzymes released into the lumen break down carbohydrates, proteins and fats.
    - Bile is released from the gallbladder into the lumen – bile salts emulsify fats to increase the surface area for digestion.
    - The small bowel is specialized for its absorptive function:
        - Approximately 6 metres in length with the mucosa forming folds increasing the surface area threefold.
        - Finger-like projections called villi increase the surface area a further tenfold:
            ○ Contain blood vessels and lymphatic vessels for absorption of nutrients.
        - Enterocytes line the small bowel:
            ○ Microvilli at the luminal surface (known as the brush border) further increase the surface area by a factor of 20.
            ○ The brush border contains enzymes to digest carbohydrate (disaccharidases) and protein (brush border and cytoplasmic peptidases).
        - Overall these adaptations increase the small bowel surface area by 600 times compared to a flat mucosa.

- Normal absorption therefore requires:
  - An intact mucosa and functioning enterocytes.
  - Normal function of the lymphatic and vascular systems.
  - Adequate pancreatic enzyme production and release.
  - Adequate bile production and release.
  - Muscles to push food along.
- Pathophysiology of malabsorption:
  - Mucosal damage: coeliac disease, Crohn's disease, radiation, Whipple's disease (see Chapter 7), tropical sprue, ischaemia, amyloidosis.
  - Pancreatic insufficiency: chronic pancreatitis, cystic fibrosis (CF), cancer of the pancreas, pancreatic resection.
  - Biliary insufficiency: primary biliary cirrhosis, biliary obstruction, biliary atresia, ileal resection (loss of circulating bile acid pool).
  - Enzyme deficiencies (intraluminal or brush border): lactase deficiency.
  - Infection: giardiasis, small intestinal bacterial overgrowth (SIBO), HIV, parasites.
  - Drug induced: cholestyramine, tetracycline, antacids, colchicine etc.
  - Reduction in small bowel length (e.g. post surgery).
  - Lymphatic obstruction: removal of concentration gradient for diffusion:
    - Lymphoma, tumours, surgery, lymphangiectasia.
  - Liver disease: reduced bile salt reuptake in the liver, reduced bile secretion.

CLINICAL FEATURES

- Varies depending on organs affected and severity of underlying disease.
- Symptoms:
  - Intestinal:
    - Diarrhoea.
    - Steatorrhoea (fatty stool).
    - Weight loss.
    - Bloating.
    - Cramping.
  - Extra-intestinal:
    - Fatigue: secondary to anaemia (reduced iron, folate, vitamin B_{12} absorption) or reduced energy absorption.
    - Dry skin/dermatitis: reduced B vitamins, niacin.
    - Thin hair.
    - Bone pain/myopathy: reduced vitamin D and calcium.
    - Bruising: reduced vitamin K.
    - Night blindness: reduced vitamin A.

- Loss of peripheral sensation: reduced vitamins B_{12} and E.
- Sore mouth: reduced vitamin B_{12} and iron.
- Examination:
  - Characteristic skin signs:
    - Casal's necklace: red/brown blistering or scaling rash around neck due to niacin (vitamin B_3) deficiency.
    - Acrodermatitis enteropathica: erythematous plaques and scaling rash sometimes with presence of vesicles due to zinc deficiency.
    - Dermatitis herpetiformis: papulovesicular symmetrical rash on elbows, knees, back, buttocks, scalp and groin due to coeliac disease.
    - Scurvy: perifollicular haemorrhages, follicular hyperkeratosis (vitamin C deficiency).
  - Muscle wasting.
  - Oedema secondary to protein deficiency.
  - Anaemia: low vitamin B_{12}, iron, folate.
  - Cheilitis/glossitis: reduced B_{12}, iron, other B vitamins.
  - Swollen gums: reduced vitamin C.
  - Peripheral neuropathy: reduced vitamin B_{12}, thiamine, vitamin E, copper.

COMPLICATIONS

- Anaemia.
- Gallstones: seen in terminal ileal disease secondary to reduced reabsorption of bile salts (supersaturation of bile with cholesterol).
- Malnutrition.
- Kidney stones: calcium oxalate stones in fat malabsorption.
- Osteoporosis.
- Weight loss.
- Malignancy: lymphoma in coeliac disease and Crohn's disease.

INVESTIGATIONS

- Blood tests:
  - Haematology: FBC, ferritin, folic acid, B_{12}, prothrombin time.
  - Chemistry: U&E, magnesium, calcium, phosphate, fat-soluble vitamins (vitamins A, D, E and K), trace elements (copper, zinc, selenium).
  - Immunology: coeliac antibodies.
- Faecal tests:
  - Parasites: e.g. Giardia, *Taenia solium*.
  - Pancreatic function: faecal elastase.
  - Calprotectin: used to detect inflammatory conditions.

Gastroenterology

- Hydrogen breath test: bacterial overgrowth, lactase deficiency.
- Small bowel imaging:
  - Barium enteroclysis/follow-through.
  - CT enteroclysis.
  - MRI enteroclysis.
- Isotope scans:
  - White cell scans: ^{99m}Tc-HMPAO (technetium 99 hexamethyl-propylamine-oxime leucocyte scan):
    - Show inflammation in the small bowel.
- Endoscopy:
  - OGD and duodenal biopsy for diagnosis of coeliac disease, Whipple's disease, tropical sprue, giardiasis.
  - Capsule endoscopy for diagnosis of Crohn's disease or coeliac disease.
- Jejunal aspiration: bacterial overgrowth and giardiasis.
- Rectal biopsy: amyloidosis.

MANAGEMENT

- Treatment of malnutrition (see Section 2.3).
- Treatment of the underlying cause.

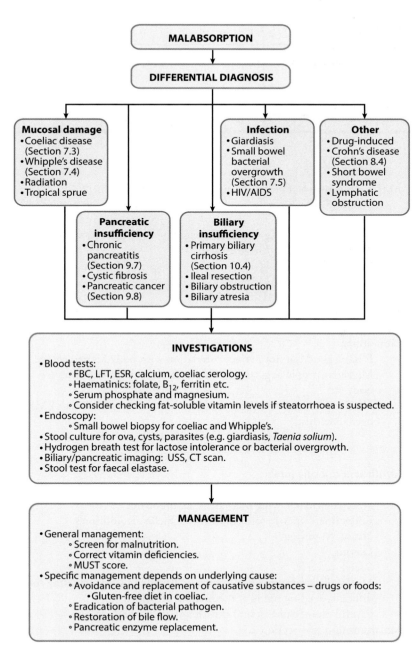

MALABSORPTION

↓

DIFFERENTIAL DIAGNOSIS

Mucosal damage
- Coeliac disease (Section 7.3)
- Whipple's disease (Section 7.4)
- Radiation
- Tropical sprue

Infection
- Giardiasis
- Small bowel bacterial overgrowth (Section 7.5)
- HIV/AIDS

Other
- Drug-induced
- Crohn's disease (Section 8.4)
- Short bowel syndrome
- Lymphatic obstruction

Pancreatic insufficiency
- Chronic pancreatitis (Section 9.7)
- Cystic fibrosis
- Pancreatic cancer (Section 9.8)

Biliary insufficiency
- Primary biliary cirrhosis (Section 10.4)
- Ileal resection
- Biliary obstruction
- Biliary atresia

INVESTIGATIONS
- Blood tests:
  - FBC, LFT, ESR, calcium, coeliac serology.
  - Haematinics: folate, B_{12}, ferritin etc.
  - Serum phosphate and magnesium.
  - Consider checking fat-soluble vitamin levels if steatorrhoea is suspected.
- Endoscopy:
  - Small bowel biopsy for coeliac and Whipple's.
- Stool culture for ova, cysts, parasites (e.g. giardiasis, *Taenia solium*).
- Hydrogen breath test for lactose intolerance or bacterial overgrowth.
- Biliary/pancreatic imaging: USS, CT scan.
- Stool test for faecal elastase.

MANAGEMENT
- General management:
  - Screen for malnutrition.
  - Correct vitamin deficiencies.
  - MUST score.
- Specific management depends on underlying cause:
  - Avoidance and replacement of causative substances – drugs or foods:
    - Gluten-free diet in coeliac.
  - Eradication of bacterial pathogen.
  - Restoration of bile flow.
  - Pancreatic enzyme replacement.

Figure 2.1 Investigation and management of malabsorption.

Gastroenterology

2.2 WEIGHT LOSS

> **MICRO-facts**
>
> Unexplained weight loss is a red flag symptom. Weight loss of more than 5% in 1 month or 10% in 6 months requires investigation.

BODY MASS INDEX

- BMI is a measure of a person's weight relative to the height:
  - Standardizes weight by height to allow easy comparison to normal range.
- It is calculated by dividing a person's weight by the height squared:
  - BMI = weight in kg/(height in m^2).
- What does it tell us?
  - Underweight: BMI <18.5.
  - Normal weight: BMI 18.5–24.9.
  - Overweight: BMI 25–29.9.
  - Obese: BMI ≥30.
- Limitations:
  - It has a good but not perfect correlation with body fat percentage.
  - Muscular people (e.g. rugby players) can have high BMI but low body fat.
  - NICE recommends using waist circumference in addition to BMI to overcome this.

PATHOPHYSIOLOGY OF WEIGHT LOSS

- Insufficient calorific intake:
  - Psychological: anorexia, depression, dementia.
  - Neurological: chewing or swallowing problems.
  - Endocrine: hyperthyroidism, diabetes mellitus, Addison's.
  - Nausea/vomiting.
  - Dieting.
  - Social: poverty.
  - Mechanical: poor mobility causing difficulty buying/preparing food or difficulty feeding self (e.g. rheumatoid arthritis).
  - Painful mouth: ulcers, oral thrush, gingivitis, oral cancers.
- Malabsorption (see Section 2.1).
- Excess use of calories/loss of tissue (catabolic state):
  - Acute infection: any sepsis.
  - Chronic infection: HIV/AIDS, TB.

- Major surgery.
- Burns.
- Malignancy.
- Chronic disease: cardiac failure, respiratory failure, renal failure, liver failure etc.

CLINICAL FEATURES

- History:
    - Low mood, poor concentration, anhedonia, sleep disorders: depression, Addison's disease.
    - Opportunistic infections: HIV/AIDS.
    - Polydipsia, thirst, polyuria: diabetes mellitus.
    - Heat intolerance, tremor, palpitations, goitre (suggests thyrotoxicosis).
    - Specific symptoms with progressive course (suggest malignancy): mass, rectal bleeding, change in bowel habit etc.
    - Steatorrhoea, diarrhoea, abdominal pain: suggests chronic pancreatitis, coeliac disease or Crohn's disease.
- Examination:
    - General examination:
        - Goitre: thyrotoxicosis.
        - Palmar/buccal pigmentation: Addison's.
        - Mouth: signs of immunosuppression (e.g. oral candidiasis, Kaposi's sarcoma).
        - Mobility: signs of rheumatoid arthritis or other joint/mobility problems.
        - Hands: signs of joint disease (e.g. rheumatoid/osteoarthritis).
        - Skin: bruising secondary to vitamin K deficiency, skin changes secondary to scurvy or other vitamin deficiencies.
    - Abdominal examination is often normal but the following may be found:
        - Enlarged liver:
            - Primary or metastatic liver tumours.
            - Secondary to hepatitis in HIV/AIDS.
        - Abdominal mass.
        - Digital rectal examination (DRE): blood/rectal mass suggests rectal tumour, fistulae in Crohn's disease, anal cancer and HIV.
    - Neurological examination:
        - Focal neurological signs due to neurological conditions (e.g. MS) or secondary to metastatic malignancy.
        - Signs of chronic neurological disease:
            - Muscle wasting and fasciculations – motor neuron disease.

Gastroenterology

COMPLICATIONS

- Malnutrition (see Section 2.3).
- Complications mainly related to underlying pathology.

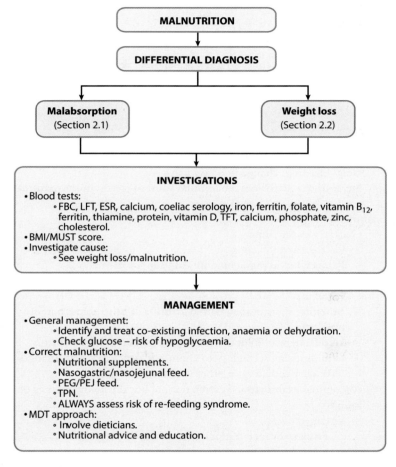

Figure 2.2 Malnutrition flow diagram.

2.3 MALNUTRITION

DEFINITION

- A state in which an imbalance in vitamin, mineral and/or nutrient intake causes adverse effects on the body:
  - Usually taken to mean under-nutrition in which there is a deficiency of particular nutrients, vitamins or minerals:
    - Can be a result of both malabsorption and weight loss.
    - Can also mean a state of over-nutrition where certain nutrients, vitamins or minerals are in excess.

EPIDEMIOLOGY

- Affects 3 million people in the UK.

MICRO-facts

Paediatric malnutrition can be broadly split into two groups, which are mainly seen in developing countries:

- Kwashiorkor (more common in older children):
  - Often an acute presentation due to concurrent stress in an individual with a reduced nutritional reserve.
  - Increased metabolic rate with increased protein and carbohydrate metabolism.
  - Protein deficiency with adequate overall calorie intake.
  - Presents with oedema, hepatomegaly, a distended abdomen (due to muscle weakness) and skin ulcers.
- Marasmus (common in infants):
  - A more chronic presentation due to starvation causing loss of subcutaneous fat and muscle.
  - Low metabolic rate with lack of energy intake.
  - Protein deficiency with inadequate overall calorie intake.
  - Presents with severe wasting, body weight less than 60% expected and loss of adipose tissue.

MICRO-print
BAPEN (The British Association for Parenteral and Enteric Nutrition) estimate that:

- 25–34% of patients admitted to hospital are at risk of malnutrition.
- 30–42% of patients admitted to care homes are at risk of malnutrition.
- 18–20% of patients admitted to mental health units are at risk of malnutrition.

RISK FACTORS

- Children:
  - Chronic illness.
  - Developmental delay.
  - Neglect.
  - Prematurity.
  - Weaning.
  - Poverty.
- Adults:
  - Chronic disease:
    - HIV/AIDS.
    - Any organ failure.
    - Chronic GI disease: Crohn's disease, coeliac disease, chronic pancreatitis.
  - Alcohol/drug addiction.
  - Chronic infections.
  - Low income.
  - Living alone.
  - Psychiatric disturbance (e.g. anorexia nervosa).
  - Malignancy.
- The elderly:
  - Loss of appetite:
    - Physiological.
    - Medication side effects: antidepressants, analgesics, antibiotics etc.
    - Nausea.
  - Chronic illness.
  - Dentures – difficulty chewing.
  - Difficulty swallowing.
  - Decreased mobility – problems shopping and cooking.
  - Poverty – less money available for food.
  - Depression.
  - Dementia.

CLINICAL FEATURES

- History:
  - Malnutrition is closely related to malabsorption and weight loss:
    - See key history points above in Sections 2.1 and 2.2.
  - Diet and nutritional intake:
    - Insufficient intake – ascertain why (social factors are important).
    - Poor nutritional content of food – may need education.

- Diarrhoea:
  - Protein-losing enteropathy: coeliac disease, Crohn's disease, chronic infections etc.
  - Small bowel disease.
  - Pancreatic disease.
- Past history:
  - Surgery – bowel resections.
  - Chronic disease.
  - Psychiatric illness.
- Examination:
  - For malabsorption signs, see Section 2.1.
  - Oedema – secondary to protein loss.
  - Muscle wasting.
  - Thinning of the hair.
  - Dry skin.
  - See Table 2.1 for specific vitamin deficiencies and their presentations.
- Malnutrition Universal Screening Tool (MUST):
  - Used to screen patients for malnutrition (see Table 2.2).

Table 2.1 **Features of vitamin deficiency**

VITAMIN	FEATURES OF DEFICIENCY
A	Xerophthalmia (dry eyes), night blindness, follicular hyperkeratosis (increased keratin in hair follicles)
B_1	Beriberi, Wernicke's encephalopathy, Korsakoff's psychosis, neuropathy
B_2	Mucosal fissuring, angular stomatitis
B_6	Neuropathy, glossitis, sideroblastic anaemia
B_{12}	Megaloblastic anaemia, neurological disorders (subacute combined degeneration of the spinal cord)
Niacin (B_3)	Pellagra (photosensitivity, dermatitis, glossitis, neurological symptoms, confusion, cardiomyopathy)
Folate (B_9)	Megaloblastic anaemia, mouth ulcers, villous atrophy
C	Scurvy (malaise, lethargy, bone pain, myalgia, shortness of breath), swollen gums
D	Rickets, osteomalacia
E	Neuropathy, anaemia
K	Coagulation defects

Gastroenterology

Table 2.2 **Malnutrition Universal Screening Tool (MUST) screen scoring**

	RANGE	SCORE
BMI	>20 18.5–20 <18.5	0 point 1 point 2 points
Recent unintentional weight loss	<5% 5–10% >10%	0 point 1 point 2 points
Acute disease effect	Risk of being unable to eat for 5 days/no food in last 5 days/acute illness	2 points if any

- Management:
  - 0 points – low risk:
    - Routine clinical care – rescreen inpatients weekly.
  - 1 point – medium risk:
    - Observe, document food intake – rescreen inpatients weekly.
  - 2 points – high risk:
    - Refer to dietician, monitor – review weekly.
    - Set goals, improve and increase nutritional intake.
- Features of vitamin deficiency (see Table 2.1).

MANAGEMENT

MICRO-facts

A major complication of artificial nutrition is re-feeding syndrome (see Section 2.3 for complications). This occurs when nutrition is given after a prolonged period of starvation. Patients must be risk assessed prior to beginning artificial nutrition.

- Treatment of any underlying cause.
- Medications causing increase in appetite: prednisolone, mirtazapine etc.
- Nutritional supplements:
  - Range of high-calorie drinks – tailored to nutritional needs (see Table 2.3).
- Artificial nutrition:
  - Immediate artificial nutrition:
    - Enteral nutrition preferred to parenteral route owing to fewer complications and maintenance of the gastrointestinal tract:
      - Nasogastric (NG) tube: passed from the nose into the stomach:
        - Nutrients passed directly into the stomach.

Table 2.3 **Nutritional requirements**

NUTRIENT	DAILY REQUIREMENT
Overall energy requirements	20–25 kcal/kg/day if healthy 30–35 kcal/kg/day if acutely ill (catabolic state)
Glucose	4–5 g/kg/day (50% of energy requirement)
Protein	0.75 g/kg/day (20% of energy requirement)
Lipid	1 g/kg/day
Sodium	100–150 mmol/day
Potassium	60–90 mmol/day
Chloride	110 mmol/day
Magnesium	9 mmol/day
Phosphate	30–40 mmol/day
Calcium	5–15 mmol/day
Water	2.5–3 litres per day

- ○ Nasojejunal (NJ) tube: passed from the nose into the jejunum:
  - ○ Can be used when the stomach is not functional (gastroparesis).
- – Parenteral nutrition:
  - ○ Total parenteral nutrition (TPN):
    - ○ Nutrients given directly into the venous blood stream usually via a PICC line (peripherally inserted central catheter).
    - ○ Indications: intestinal obstruction, ileus, short bowel syndrome etc.
- Long-term artificial nutrition:
  - – Percutaneous endoscopic gastrostomy (PEG):
    - ○ Endoscopically placed port inserted through anterior abdominal wall allows direct insertion of food into the stomach.
  - – Percutaneous endoscopic jejunostomy (PEJ):
    - ○ Similar to a PEG but used if the stomach is not functional (e.g. gastroparesis).
  - – Surgical gastrostomy/jejunostomy:
    - ○ Feeding ports can be inserted surgically usually when there is concurrent abdominal surgery.
  - – Total parenteral nutrition (as above).

Gastroenterology

> **MICRO-reference**
> NICE guidelines on nutrition support in adults: http://pathways.nice.
> org.uk/pathways/nutrition-support-in-adults

COMPLICATIONS

- Complications of malnutrition:
  - Impaired immune function.
  - Impaired wound healing.
  - Muscle wasting: increased risk of falls.
  - Impaired renal function.
  - Reduction in fertility.
  - Depression.
  - Impaired cardiac function.
  - Complications for children and adolescents:
    - Growth failure.
    - Delayed puberty.
    - Lower peak bone mass density and consequent increased risk of osteoporosis later in life.
    - Rickets.
    - Impaired intellectual development.
- Complications of artificial nutrition:
  - Re-feeding syndrome:
    - Occurs when feeding is recommenced after a period of malnutrition.
    - Risk factors for re-feeding syndrome as set out in NICE clinical guideline 32 (see Table 2.4):

Table 2.4 **Risk factors for re-feeding syndrome**

ONE OR MORE OF	TWO OR MORE OF
BMI <16 kg/m²	BMI <18.5 kg/m²
Unintentional weight loss >15% in the last 3–6 months	Unintentional weight loss >10% in the last 3–6 months
Little or no nutritional intake for more than 10 days	Little or no nutritional intake for more than 5 days
Low levels of potassium, phosphate or magnesium prior to feeding	A history of alcohol abuse or drugs including insulin, chemotherapy, antacids or diuretics

Gastroenterology

- During starvation the body enters a catabolic state:
  - Low carbohydrate intake results in low insulin secretion.
  - Insulin aids uptake of intracellular ions, such as phosphate, magnesium and potassium into cells.
  - Low insulin levels lead to reduced intracellular uptake and depletion of intracellular phosphate stores.
  - Beginning feeding increases insulin levels – increases cellular phosphate uptake, as well as the uptake of potassium and magnesium.
  - Phosphate also used in the glycolytic pathway and protein synthesis.
  - Results in low serum phosphate levels (usually within 4 days) and also low potassium and magnesium levels.
  - Rhabdomyolysis, respiratory insufficiency, arrhythmias, hypotension, seizures, leukocyte dysfunction, coma and sudden death can all occur.
  - Risk must be assessed before beginning artificial nutrition.
- Management:
  - Re-introduce feeding slowly: Initially no more than 10–15 kcal/kg/day in high-risk patients.
  - Check phosphate, magnesium and potassium levels prior to re-feeding, correct as needed and monitor daily initially during re-feeding.
  - Use of parenteral B vitamins (Pabrinex) prevents deficiency – used in co-enzymes during glycolysis.
- Complications of a PEG:
  - General – serious complications occur in 0.5–8%.
    - Immediate: bleeding, wound infection, chest infection etc.
    - Later: aspiration, dislodging of PEG, blockage, wound infection, diarrhoea, oesophagitis.
  - PEG tubes can fall out:
    - Should be replaced as soon as possible as the orifice starts to close within 30 minutes.
    - If replacement is not available, a similar gauge (usually 16 French) Foley catheter should be inserted temporarily.
  - Blockage:
    - PEG tubes should be flushed before and after use with water.
    - Tubes commonly become blocked with crushed medications or protein precipitation from feeds.
    - Proprietary preparations are available to unblock tubes.
    - Sodium bicarbonate ± pancreatic enzymes often works if other solutions are not available.

- Complications of TPN:
  - Line sepsis/thrombosis.
  - Not physiological – risk of muscle hypertrophy, hyperglycaemia and liver damage.

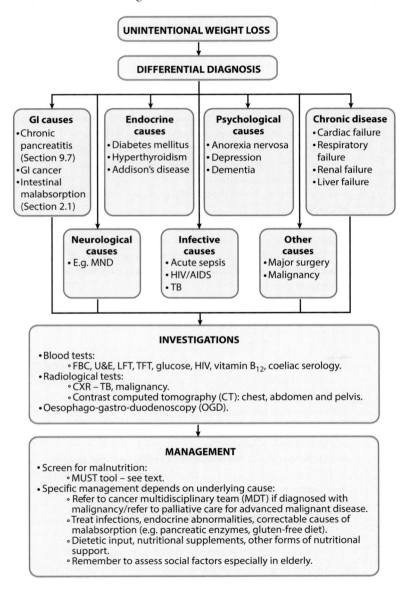

Figure 2.3 Investigation and management of weight loss.

MICRO-case

An elderly man is brought to the ED after being found wandering in the street outside his house. He is confused and appears thin and unkempt. A review of the previous notes reveals he has had no previous admissions in the last 3 years. At a previous admission, he was noted to be slightly confused with a Mini-Mental State Examination (MMSE) score of 24 out of 30. After this admission, he was discharged home with his wife. After discussion with the patient's GP, it becomes clear that the patient's wife died some 18 months previously. The GP has not seen the patient for many months. It seems that there has been very little support since his wife died and he has been struggling to care for himself.

He is transferred to the Care of the Elderly ward once a septic screen has been carried out to rule out infection-induced delirium. The patient's BMI is found to be only 18.1, so the team is keen to improve this patient's nutritional status and ask for a dietician review. The dietician calculates the patient's MUST score. It is felt that due to a poor nutritional intake for a prolonged period of time and a low BMI, this patient is at risk of re-feeding syndrome. Blood tests are taken for phosphate, magnesium and potassium before initiation of feeding and arranged daily thereafter. Haematinics are also requested to rule out folic acid deficiency.

Over the first few days, it is noted that the patient's oral intake is poor and his confusion means he is struggling to understand the importance of increasing his intake. It is decided that he would benefit from NG tube feeding. Despite pulling his NG tube out on two occasions, he improves over the following weeks.

His confusion improves although a formal diagnosis of Alzheimer's disease is made. The decision is made that the patient is now medically fit and discharge planning begins. It is felt that he is unable to care for himself, and so arrangements are made for him to move into a care home where he can be supported with his activities of daily living.

Key points:

- Malnutrition is a common problem, not just on a gastroenterology ward, but also in other areas of healthcare:
  - The MUST score predicts a patient's risk of malnutrition.
- Folic acid deficiency is common in the elderly and those in residential care.
- Re-feeding syndrome occurs when feeding is restarted after a period of poor nutritional intake.
- Monitoring of phosphate, magnesium and potassium is vital.
- Oral intake with supplements should be encouraged as a first measure in most patients.
- Artificial nutrition may be appropriate in some patients if oral intake remains poor but comes with added risk.

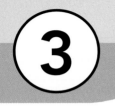

Common colonic presentations

3.1 DIARRHOEA

DEFINITION

- Abnormal passage of loose motions more than three times per day and/or a quantity of stool greater than 200 g/day.
- Divided into acute and chronic diarrhoea:
    - Acute diarrhoea: usually up to a 2-week period but could occasionally continue for 4 weeks.
    - Chronic diarrhoea: persisting symptoms of diarrhoea lasting for more than 4 weeks.

AETIOLOGY

- See Figure 3.1 for causes of acute and chronic diarrhoea.

PATHOPHYSIOLOGY

- Osmotic diarrhoea:
    - Ingestion of poorly absorbed, osmotically active anions, cations or sugars resulting in reversal of the fluid balance from absorption to secretion (i.e. mannitol, lactose).
- Secretory diarrhoea:
    - Activation of intestinal ion secretion or blockage of absorptive pathways secondary to a variety of agents (i.e. bacterial exotoxins, hormones, drugs).
    - Loss of surface area impairing fluid and electrolyte absorption (e.g. in coeliac disease, surgical resection, inflammatory bowel disease).
    - Inflammatory diarrhoea caused by disruption of mucosal integrity (e.g. inflammatory bowel disease, amoebiasis).
- Diarrhoea of infectious cause:
    - Same as for secretory diarrhoea.
    - Destruction of the intestinal epithelial cells by the offending organism causing passage of blood and mucus and preventing effective absorption.

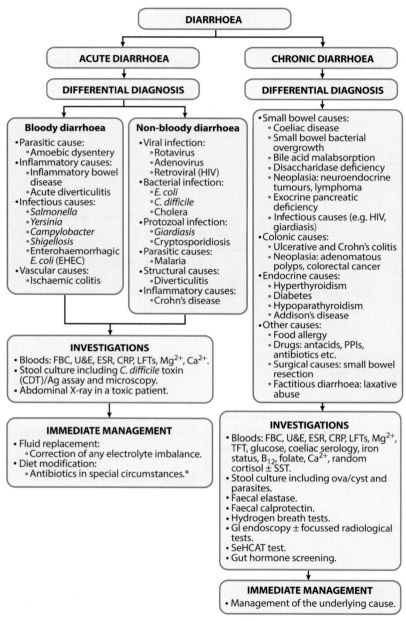

Figure 3.1 Investigations and management of diarrhoea.

* Locke T, Keat S, Mackinnon R. *Microbiology and Infectious Diseases on the Move.* London: Hodder Arnold Publishing; 2012. pp. 128–133.

Gastroenterology

- Diarrhoea due to abnormal intestinal motility:
  - Accelerated transit time interfering with water absorption (e.g. IBS, diabetes mellitus).
  - Delayed transit time (resulting in bacterial overgrowth).

CLINICAL FEATURES

- History:
  - Timing and frequency:
    - Duration of diarrhoea (acute versus chronic).
    - Nocturnal diarrhoea is suggestive of an organic cause.
  - Consistency, smell, colour and volume:
    - Large volume watery diarrhoea is more suggestive of small bowel origin (giardiasis).
    - Profuse diarrhoea is suggestive of secretory aetiology (cholera).
    - Smaller volume mucoid/bloody diarrhoea is more suggestive of large bowel origin (*Entamoeba histolytica*, *Clostridium difficile*).
    - Foul-smelling, yellow stool that floats is suggestive of steatorrhoea (pancreatic insufficiency).
  - Associated symptoms:
    - Vomiting (rotavirus infection).
    - Weight loss (Crohn's disease, hyperthyroidism, malignancy).
    - Abdominal pain (inflammatory bowel disease, IBS, infectious diarrhoea).
    - Rectal bleeding: infectious and inflammatory causes (shigellosis, ulcerative colitis, diverticular disease).
  - Other history:
    - Travel and food history:
      - ○ Enterotoxicogenic *Escherichia coli* is the most common cause of traveller's diarrhoea.
      - ○ Campylobacter infection is associated with poultry consumption as well as contact with pets (e.g. puppies).
    - Animal contact (salmonellosis).
    - Premorbid factors (*C. difficile* infection in hospitalized patients and/or recent antibiotic use).
- Examination:
  - General signs of dehydration:
    - Mild–moderate dehydration: restless, thirsty, tachycardia, low urine output, dry mucus membrane, cool extremities, poor skin turgor.
    - Severe dehydration: lethargic/comatose, tachy/bradycardia, absent urine output, dry mucus membranes, poor skin turgor, cold extremities.
  - Fever (infective or inflammatory causes).
  - Abdominal tenderness ± signs of peritonitis.

Gastroenterology

INVESTIGATIONS

- Acute diarrhoea:
  - Investigate in prolonged cases with any of the following features:
    - Fever.
    - Bloody diarrhoea.
    - Immunocompromised host.
    - Recent antibiotic use.
    - Elderly patient.
  - See Figure 3.1 for immediate investigations.
- Chronic diarrhoea:
  - See Figure 3.1 for immediate investigations.
  - If the history is suggestive of IBS (as per Rome III criteria), no further investigation is required.

> **MICRO-reference**
> See the Rome III diagnostic criteria for further information on the classification of irritable bowel syndrome: http://www.romecriteria.org/assets/pdf/19_RomeIII_apA_885-898.pdf

COMPLICATIONS

- Toxic megacolon.
- Peritonitis.
- Malabsorption.
- Dehydration/acute kidney injury.
- Electrolyte imbalance.
- Malignancy (long-standing inflammatory bowel disease, coeliac disease).

> **MICRO-reference**
> See the WGO guidelines for further information on the classification and management of dehydration in children and adults with diarrhoea: http://www.worldgastroenterology.org/assets/export/userfiles/Acute%20Diarrhea_long_FINAL_120604.pdf

Gastroenterology

MICRO-facts

Management of non-surgical dehydration (WHO guideline)
- No dehydration (<3% water loss in adults): encourage normal diet and fluids.
- Mild/moderate dehydration (3–9% water loss in adults): oral rehydration solution (ORS)* 30–80 mL/hr; NG tube hydration if not tolerated orally.†
- Severe hydration (>9% water loss in adults): IV hydration 20 mL/hr initially and reassess.

---

* ORS consists of sodium (75 mmol/L), chloride (65 mmol/L), anhydrous glucose (75 mmol/L), potassium (20 mmol/L) and trisodium citrate (10 mmol/L) with a total osmolarity of 245 mmol/L.
† Vomiting is not a contraindication to oral therapy as long as net intake is more than output.

3.2 CONSTIPATION

DEFINITION

- Must include two or more of the following in at least 25% of defaecations (as per the Rome III criteria):
  - Straining.
  - Hard stools.
  - Feeling of incomplete evacuation.
  - Sensation of anorectal blockage.
  - Manual manoeuvres to facilitate evacuation.
  - Less than three bowel movements per week.
- Symptoms must be present for at least 6 months with at least two of the Rome III criteria having been met for the past 3 months for a diagnosis to be made.

AETIOLOGY

- See Figure 3.2 for causes of constipation.

PATHOPHYSIOLOGY

- Slow-transit constipation (colonic inertia): slow passage of stool throughout the colon due to slow or uncoordinated peristalsis:
  - Can be primary or secondary:
    - Primary: functional constipation.
    - Secondary:
      - Endocrine disorders (hypothyroidism, diabetes).

Gastroenterology

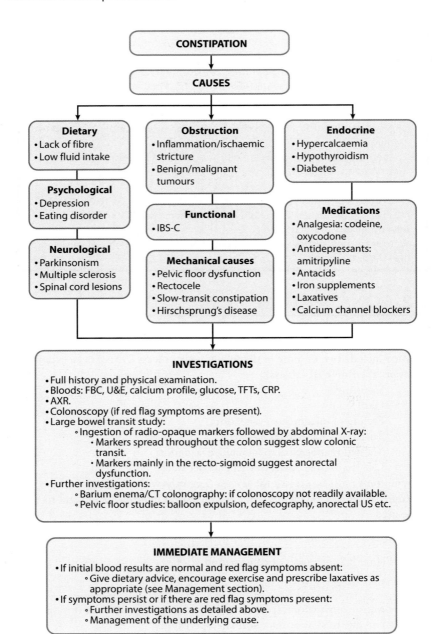

CONSTIPATION

CAUSES

Dietary
• Lack of fibre
• Low fluid intake

Psychological
• Depression
• Eating disorder

Neurological
• Parkinsonism
• Multiple sclerosis
• Spinal cord lesions

Obstruction
• Inflammation/ischaemic stricture
• Benign/malignant tumours

Functional
• IBS-C

Mechanical causes
• Pelvic floor dysfunction
• Rectocele
• Slow-transit constipation
• Hirschsprung's disease

Endocrine
• Hypercalcaemia
• Hypothyroidism
• Diabetes

Medications
• Analgesia: codeine, oxycodone
• Antidepressants: amitripyline
• Antacids
• Iron supplements
• Laxatives
• Calcium channel blockers

INVESTIGATIONS
• Full history and physical examination.
• Bloods: FBC, U&E, calcium profile, glucose, TFTs, CRP.
• AXR.
• Colonoscopy (if red flag symptoms are present).
• Large bowel transit study:
  ○ Ingestion of radio-opaque markers followed by abdominal X-ray:
    · Markers spread throughout the colon suggest slow colonic transit.
    · Markers mainly in the recto-sigmoid suggest anorectal dysfunction.
• Further investigations:
  ○ Barium enema/CT colonography: if colonoscopy not readily available.
  ○ Pelvic floor studies: balloon expulsion, defecography, anorectal US etc.

IMMEDIATE MANAGEMENT
• If initial blood results are normal and red flag symptoms absent:
  ○ Give dietary advice, encourage exercise and prescribe laxatives as appropriate (see Management section).
• If symptoms persist or if there are red flag symptoms present:
  ○ Further investigations as detailed above.
  ○ Management of the underlying cause.

Figure 3.2 Constipation flow diagram.

Gastroenterology

- ○ Drug related (opioids, antihypertensives, anticholinergics).
- ○ Electrolyte abnormalities (hypokalaemia, hypercalcaemia).
- ○ Neurological disorders (multiple sclerosis, Hirschsprung's disease).
- ○ Others (systemic sclerosis, amyloidosis).
- ● Pelvic floor dysfunction (outlet obstruction): difficulty passing stool that has been accumulated in the rectum:
  - Can be due to inadequate relaxation/incoordination of puborectalis muscle or external anal sphincter during defaecation.
  - Rectocele can be contributory or the main cause of constipation.

CLINICAL FEATURES

- ● As per Rome III criteria for diagnosis of functional constipation (see Section 3.1).
- ● History:
  - Abdominal bloating.
  - Overflow diarrhoea.
  - Low back pain.
  - Pain on defaecation.
  - Tenesmus.
- ● Red flag symptoms necessitating colonic investigation:
  - Persistent rectal bleeding without rectal signs (age >60 years).
  - Change of bowel habit to looser stools/increased frequency for 6 weeks in patients over 60.
  - Change of bowel habit to looser stools/increased frequency and rectal bleeding.
  - Palpable right iliac fossa mass.
  - Palpable rectal mass.
  - Unexplained iron deficiency anaemia <110 g/L men, <100 g/L in non-menstruating women.

INVESTIGATIONS

Only required in a minority of patients with severe and intractable symptoms, or in patients exhibiting red flag symptoms.
- ● See Figure 3.2 for investigations for constipation.

MANAGEMENT

- ● Lifestyle advice:
  - Dietary advice including high fibre and fluid intake:
    - – Increase gradually to 25 g of fibre per day.
  - Encourage regular exercise.
  - Psychological counselling as required.
  - Pelvic floor retraining with biofeedback and muscle relaxation used in pelvic floor dysfunction.

Gastroenterology

- Pharmacological intervention:
  - Laxatives:
    - Bulk-forming laxatives: ispaghula husk, methylcellulose, bran.
    - Osmotic laxatives: lactulose, milk of magnesia, polyethylene glycol.
    - Stool softeners: docusate sodium, mineral oil, glycerine suppositories.
    - Stimulant laxatives: castor oil, senna.
    - Prokinetic laxatives: prucalopride.
- Surgical intervention:
  - Indicated in cases of retractable slow-transit constipation unassociated with obstructed defaecation:
    - Total colectomy with ileorectal anastomosis.
    - Antegrade colonic enema (ACE) procedure: a button stoma is made in the caecum to allow installation of daily water enemas.

3.3 RECTAL BLEEDING (LOWER GI BLEEDING)

DEFINITION

- Bleeding distal to the ligament of Treitz.

AETIOLOGY

- See Figure 3.3 for the differential diagnosis of rectal bleeding.

CLINICAL FEATURES

- History:
  - Features of the bleeding:
    - Blood limited to the toilet paper or to the surface of the formed stool: perianal source (haemorrhoids, fissure) likely.
    - Anal pruritis and pain on defaecation: anal source of bleeding likely.
  - Associated symptoms:
    - Fever (inflammatory bowel disease, diverticulitis).
    - Weight loss (malignancy, inflammatory bowel disease).
    - Abdominal pain (diverticulitis, malignancy, IBD).
  - Comorbidities:
    - Liver disease/cirrhosis.
    - Coagulopathy.
    - Inflammatory bowel disease.
    - Malignancy (colorectal cancer).
    - Peptic ulcer disease.
    - Diverticular disease.
    - Heart failure and atrial fibrillation (ischaemic colitis).

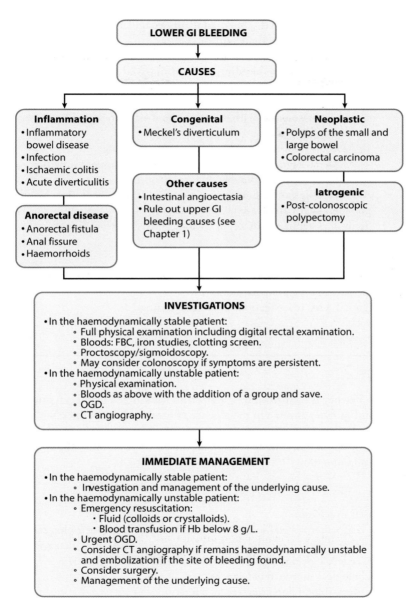

Figure 3.3 Investigations and management of lower GI bleeding.

- Drug history (NSAIDs, nicorandil, anticoagulation therapy).
- Travel history (infectious causes).
- Examination:
  - Rectal examination: bleeding varies from trivial haematochezia to massive haemorrhage:
    - Bright red bleeding per rectum: usually left colon pathology but can also occur with more proximal GI pathology if massive bleeding.
    - Maroon stool: suggestive of right colon pathology.
    - Melaena: suggestive of caecal, small bowel or upper GI pathology.
  - Abdominal tenderness/mass.
  - Associated signs of haemodynamic instability and shock (low blood pressure, tachycardia, tachypnoea etc.).
  - Signs of anaemia (common in chronic per rectum bleeding).

INVESTIGATIONS

- Dependent upon the severity, volume and frequency of the bleeding, along with the patient's haemodynamic status.
- See Figure 3.3 for investigations of rectal bleeding.

3.4 IRON DEFICIENCY ANAEMIA

DEFINITION

- Iron deficiency is confirmed by a low serum ferritin, red blood cell microcytosis and/or hypochromia in the absence of haemoglobinopathies:
  - As ferritin is an acute-phase protein, serum levels may be normal or even high in iron deficiency anaemia if there is concomitant inflammation.

RISK FACTORS

- Increased iron loss:
  - Gastroenterological source (colorectal cancer, gastro-oesophageal cancer, peptic ulcer disease, NSAID use with associated ulceration).
  - Gynaecological source (menstruation, endometrial cancer).
  - Urological source (renal cancer).
  - Others (blood donation, recent surgery).
- Decreased iron intake or absorption:
  - Malabsorption (coeliac disease, Crohn's disease).
  - Inadequate dietary intake (vegetarian, old age).
  - Post total/partial gastric bypass surgery.
  - Chronic *Helicobacter pylori* gastritis causing gastric atrophy.

- Increased iron demand:
  - Pregnancy.
  - Breast feeding.
  - Rapid growth in infancy or adolescence.

CLINICAL FEATURES

- History:
  - Fatigue.
  - Rectal bleeding.
  - Poor oral intake.
  - Dyspepsia.
  - Shortness of breath.
  - Palpitations.
  - Headache.
  - Hair loss.
  - Sore tongue (glossitis).
  - Poor concentration.
  - Pica (craving for non-nutritive substances like ice, paint, sand, clay etc.).
  - Symptoms of acute or chronic bleeding (melaena, haematemesis, haematuria, haemoptysis, menorrhagia, chronic epistaxis).
  - Family history of GI cancer (Osler–Weber–Rendu syndrome).
- Examination:
  - Brittle nails.
  - Weight loss (malignancy).
  - Epigastric tenderness.
  - Oral telangiectasia.
  - Abdominal mass.
  - 'Chicken skin' of neck (pseudoxanthoma elasticum).

AETIOLOGY

- See Figure 3.4 for causes of iron deficiency anaemia.

DIFFERENTIAL DIAGNOSIS

- Anaemia of chronic disease.
- Sideroblastic anaemia.
- Haemoglobinopathies (e.g. thalassaemia).

> **MICRO-reference**
> See the British Society of Gastroenterology (BSG) guideline on the management of iron deficiency anaemia: http://www.bsg.org.uk/images/stories/docs/clinical/guidelines/sbn/bsg_ida_2011.pdf

Gastroenterology

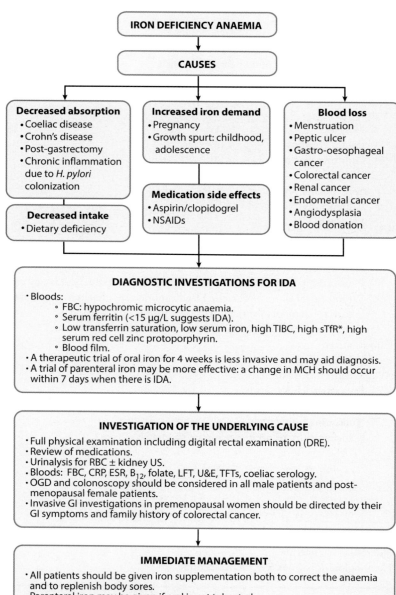

IRON DEFICIENCY ANAEMIA

↓

CAUSES

Decreased absorption
- Coeliac disease
- Crohn's disease
- Post-gastrectomy
- Chronic inflammation due to *H. pylori* colonization

Decreased intake
- Dietary deficiency

Increased iron demand
- Pregnancy
- Growth spurt: childhood, adolescence

Medication side effects
- Aspirin/clopidogrel
- NSAIDs

Blood loss
- Menstruation
- Peptic ulcer
- Gastro-oesophageal cancer
- Colorectal cancer
- Renal cancer
- Endometrial cancer
- Angiodysplasia
- Blood donation

DIAGNOSTIC INVESTIGATIONS FOR IDA
- Bloods:
  - FBC: hypochromic microcytic anaemia.
  - Serum ferritin (<15 µg/L suggests IDA).
  - Low transferrin saturation, low serum iron, high TIBC, high sTfR*, high serum red cell zinc protoporphyrin.
  - Blood film.
- A therapeutic trial of oral iron for 4 weeks is less invasive and may aid diagnosis.
- A trial of parenteral iron may be more effective: a change in MCH should occur within 7 days when there is IDA.

INVESTIGATION OF THE UNDERLYING CAUSE
- Full physical examination including digital rectal examination (DRE).
- Review of medications.
- Urinalysis for RBC ± kidney US.
- Bloods: FBC, CRP, ESR, B_{12}, folate, LFT, U&E, TFTs, coeliac serology.
- OGD and colonoscopy should be considered in all male patients and post-menopausal female patients.
- Invasive GI investigations in premenopausal women should be directed by their GI symptoms and family history of colorectal cancer.

IMMEDIATE MANAGEMENT
- All patients should be given iron supplementation both to correct the anaemia and to replenish body sores.
- Parenteral iron may be given if oral is not tolerated.

* Soluble transferrin receptor (sTfR) is a truncated monomer of its tissue receptor for transferrin; a high sTfR level corresponds with tissue iron deficiency as well as bone marrow erythropoietic activity (haemolysis or ineffective erythropoiesis).

Figure 3.4 Iron deficiency anaemia flow diagram.

3.5 ABDOMINAL PAIN

DEFINITION

- May be classified as acute or chronic:
    - Acute abdominal pain occurs suddenly and is commonly associated with physiological insults.
    - Chronic abdominal pain may be present for several months.

AETIOLOGY

- See Figure 3.5 for causes of abdominal pain.

PATHOPHYSIOLOGY

- Results from stimulation of receptors specific for thermal, mechanical or chemical stimuli.
- Can be characterized as somatic or visceral:
    - Visceral pain originates from the visceral peritoneum and intra-abdominal organs.
    - Somatic pain originates from the parietal peritoneum and abdominal wall.

CLINICAL FEATURES

- History:
    - Features of the abdominal pain:
        - Onset, location, intensity, quality, timing, radiation and duration (severe central abdominal pain which subsequently localizes to the right iliac fossa is typical of appendicitis).
        - Alleviating or aggravating factors (lack of movement in peritonitis, inability to stay still in renal colic).
    - Associated symptoms:
        - Fever (infective causes, e.g. liver abscess).
        - Syncope or pre-syncope (leaking aortic aneurysm).
        - Persistent vomiting (bowel obstruction).
        - GI blood loss (diverticulitis).
        - Constipation (bowel obstruction).
- Examination:
    - Vital signs (beware of indicators of haemodynamic instability).
    - Abdominal mass.
    - Bowel sounds (check for bruit).
    - Murphy's sign for cholecystitis (tenderness below the costal margin at the right mid-clavicular line during inspiration).

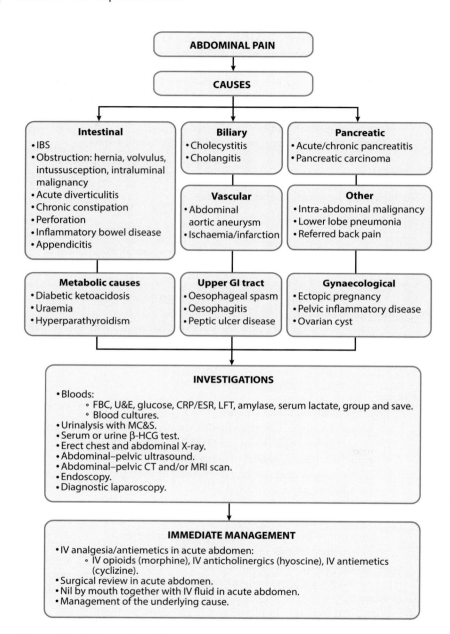

Figure 3.5 Abdominal pain flow diagram.

- McBurney's sign for appendicitis (deep tenderness at McBurney's point, which is located one-third of the distance in a hypothetical line from the right anterior superior iliac spine to the umbilicus).
- Psoas sign for appendicitis (abdominal tenderness during passive hyperextension of the right thigh while the patient is on left lateral recumbent position).
- Carnett's sign in abdominal wall pain (worsening or unchanged abdominal pain while tensing the abdominal wall muscles on supine position by lifting the shoulders or legs off the examining table).
- Rectal examination (retrocaecal appendicitis, faecal impaction, rectal mass, fresh blood/melaena).
- Pelvic examination (adnexal tenderness, vaginal discharge, testicular torsion).
- Examination of other systems:
  - Respiratory examination (lower lobe pneumonia).
  - Cardiovascular examination (atrial fibrillation).

INVESTIGATIONS

- Should be tailored according to the differential diagnosis.
- See Figure 3.5 for a full list of investigations.

MANAGEMENT

- Management of the underlying cause.
- Where diagnosis cannot be made, a fundamental aspect of management is watchful waiting with repeated questioning and reassessment of clinical course that often elucidates the true nature of the illness:
  - In most instances of acute abdominal pain, a diagnosis is readily established.
  - Success is not so frequent in patients with chronic abdominal pain.

MICRO-case

A 38-year-old chef is a lifelong smoker and has been drinking on average 70 units of alcohol per week since his second divorce 8 years ago. He had a hospital admission for acute pancreatitis 4 years ago and was warned about the adverse effects of alcohol and smoking. He intermittently stopped drinking alcohol for several months on two occasions but unfortunately returned due to complicated family dynamics.

continued...

Gastroenterology

continued...

He made an appointment with his GP due to ongoing gradual weight loss of 9 kg over the past 6 months despite adhering to a high-calorie diet. During the consultation, he mentions that he has been having looser and more frequent bowel motions recently. On direct questioning, he describes his motions as pale malodorous stools, which tend to float on top of the toilet water.

On examination, he looks thin with a BMI of 19. There is no peripheral lymphadenopathy and no peripheral signs of chronic liver disease. He has slight tenderness over the epigastric region of the abdomen, but no masses are palpable. The rest of the examination is unremarkable.

Blood results show normal FBC, U&Es, IgGs, tTG/EMAs, CRP and ESR. LFTs are normal apart from a raised γGT of 84 U/L. HIV serology is negative. Stool culture is negative. Stool faecal pancreatic elastase is 35 μg/g of stool (normal >200 μg/g of stool). He is also sent for an urgent chest X-ray, which is normal and a CT scan of his abdomen, which reveals granular pancreatic calcification with several small pseudocysts suggestive of chronic pancreatitis.

He is put on pancreatin (Creon) with rapid resolution of symptoms and gradual weight gain over the following months. He is also strongly advised against alcohol use and smoking in order to minimize the risk of ongoing pancreatic damage.

Key points:

- Steatorrhoea is a result of fat malabsorption usually due to pancreatic or small bowel disease owing to reduction in the enzymes responsible for fat absorption.
- CT abdomen with pancreatic protocol should be considered in any patients with a significant weight loss and a background of heavy alcohol use and pancreatitis to exclude pancreatic malignancy.
- Faecal pancreatic elastase is only abnormal in severe pancreatic insufficiency (more than 75% exocrine failure) and hence a normal result does not exclude pancreatic insufficiency. An empirical trial of pancreatin therapy may be indicated following initial investigations.

Supplemental pancreatic enzymes are inactivated by gastric acid and are best taken with food. Acid secretion can be reduced using drugs such as ranitidine. Pancreatic enzymes are taken with snacks and every meal. The dose is titrated according to stool appearance, frequency and consistency.

Gastroenterology

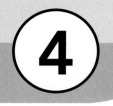

4 Common liver presentations

4.1 JAUNDICE

- Clinically detectable when plasma bilirubin exceeds 50 μmol/L.
- Subclinical jaundice is defined as plasma bilirubin >20 μmol/L.
- Can be divided into pre-hepatic, hepatic and post-hepatic causes.

PATHOPHYSIOLOGY

- Jaundice occurs when plasma bilirubin levels build up to exceed a certain threshold (see above).
- Haemoglobin and myoglobin are broken down into biliverdin and then reduced further to bilirubin in the reticuloendothelial cells of the bone marrow and spleen.
- Bilirubin is water insoluble and is transported to the liver in plasma bound to albumin.
- Bilirubin is conjugated within hepatocytes via the enzyme Uridine 5′-diphospho-glucuronyltransferase to bilirubin mono- and diglucuronides.
- Conjugated bilirubin is water soluble and is actively excreted into the hepatic canaliculi and via the bile ducts into the duodenum.
- Bilirubin is hydrolyzed by bacteria in the distal ileum and colon forming unconjugated bilirubin which is then reduced to colourless urobilinogen.
- Approximately 80–90% of urobilinogen is then excreted in faeces unchanged, or as an orange derivative called urobilin.
- The remainder is passively absorbed and transported via portal blood flow to the liver. A small amount bypasses the liver and is excreted in the urine.

AETIOLOGY

Pre-hepatic jaundice:
- Characterized by an increased serum unconjugated bilirubin with the rest of the liver function tests (LFTs) being normal:
    - Increased bilirubin production due to excessive haemolysis (see Figure 4.2 for haemolytic causes).
    - Decreased bilirubin uptake: drugs (e.g. rifampicin).

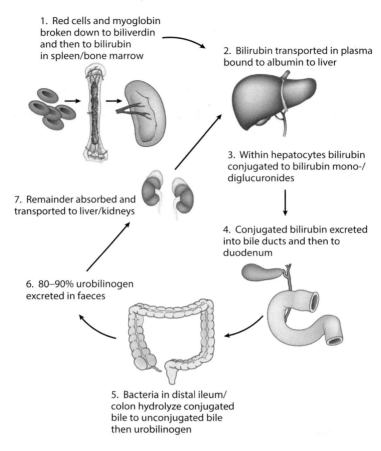

1. Red cells and myoglobin broken down to biliverdin and then to bilirubin in spleen/bone marrow

2. Bilirubin transported in plasma bound to albumin to liver

3. Within hepatocytes bilirubin conjugated to bilirubin mono-/diglucuronides

7. Remainder absorbed and transported to liver/kidneys

4. Conjugated bilirubin excreted into bile ducts and then to duodenum

6. 80–90% urobilinogen excreted in faeces

5. Bacteria in distal ileum/colon hydrolyze conjugated bile to unconjugated bile then urobilinogen

Figure 4.1 Mechanism of bilirubin breakdown.

- Intrahepatic cholestasis:
  - Due to any mechanism which damages the hepatocytes, leading to failure of metabolism/excretion of bilirubin (see Figure 4.2 for hepatic causes).
  - Decreased bilirubin conjugation causing an isolated rise in serum unconjugated bilirubin:
    - Gilbert's syndrome:
      - ○ Autosomal dominant condition resulting in impaired bilirubin conjugation.
    - Crigler–Najjar syndrome:
      - ○ Rare conditions associated with other mutations in UDP-glucuronyltransferase.

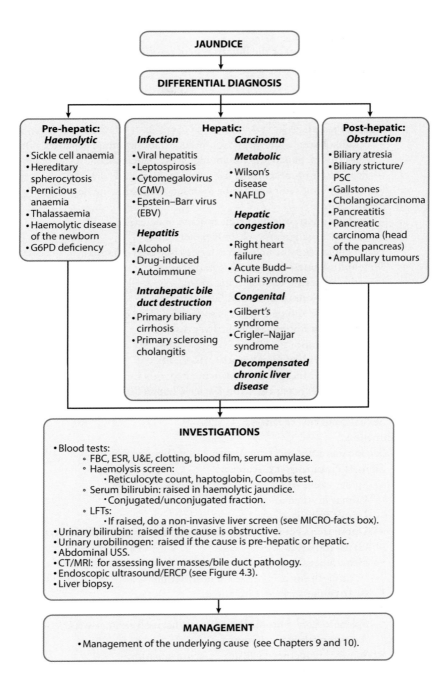

Figure 4.2 Jaundice investigations and management.

- Post-hepatic cholestasis:
  - Due to obstruction of the biliary system resulting in decreased excretion of bilirubin into the gut (see Figure 4.2 for obstructive causes).

CLINICAL FEATURES

- History:
  - Onset of jaundice:
    - Sudden onset: acute viral/drug-induced/autoimmune hepatitis, bile duct stones, pancreatic carcinoma, acute pancreatitis.
    - Progressive onset: chronic liver disease, metastatic disease.
  - Prodromal viral symptoms prior to onset: suggests acute hepatitis.
  - Pain:
    - Sudden onset: bile duct stones, acute pancreatitis.
    - Chronic: malignancy, chronic pancreatitis.
  - Fever: cholangitis (usually secondary to bile duct stones).
  - Weight loss: carcinoma, chronic pancreatitis.
  - Pruritis: suggestive of cholestatic cause.
  - Change in colour of urine and faeces:
    - Dark urine and pale faeces is suggestive of an obstructive cause.
  - Alcohol consumption: alcoholic liver disease.
  - Recent medication.
  - Drug abuse: risk of viral hepatitis (B, C, D).
  - Foreign travel: increased risk of acute hepatitis transmission in endemic areas (hepatitis A and E) (see Chapter 10).
  - Past blood transfusions (hepatitis B, C, D).
  - Sexual contacts (hepatitis B, C, D).
- Examination:
  - Sclerae (jaundice most commonly visible here first).
  - Signs of chronic liver disease:
    - Spider naevi.
    - Palmar erythema.
    - Leuconychia.
    - Dupuytren's contracture: fixed flexion deformity of the fingers.
    - Gynaecomastia.
    - Hepatomegaly:
      ○ Smooth surface: hepatitis, obstruction.
      ○ Irregular surface: carcinoma.
      ○ Tender: hepatitis.
    - Splenomegaly: chronic liver disease, haemolytic anaemias.
    - Ascites: cirrhosis, carcinoma.
  - Abdominal tenderness: gallstones, acute hepatitis.
  - Fever: cholangitis.
  - Pruritis: suggested by small scratches on the body.

COMPLICATIONS

- Kernicterus:
  - Complication of neonatal jaundice/congenital hyperbilirubinaemias:
    - In neonates, the blood–brain barrier is more permeable, allowing unconjugated bilirubin to be deposited in the basal ganglia.
    - May result in deafness, visual defects, spasticity and brain damage.
    - Management is with early phototherapy or exchange transfusion.
- Cholangitis:
  - Infection of bile usually due to an obstructed biliary system.
- Malabsorption:
  - Decreased excretion of bile causes malabsorption of fat-soluble vitamins (vitamins A, D, E and K).
- Hepatic failure.
- Renal failure.
- Malignancy:
  - Hepatocellular carcinoma complicating cirrhosis.
  - Cholangiocarcinoma complicating primary sclerosing cholangitis.

MICRO-facts

Non-invasive liver screen:

- Autoantibodies (anti-nuclear, anti-mitochondrial, P-ANCA, anti-smooth muscle, anti-LKM)
- Viral hepatitis serology (A, B, C)
- Ferritin/transferrin saturation
- α-1 Antitrypsin
- Fasting blood glucose
- Coeliac screen (anti-tTG)
- Caeruloplasmin/24-hour urinary copper
- Immunoglobulins
- Abdominal USS
- Alpha-fetoprotein

Gastroenterology

4.2 LIVER FAILURE

DEFINITION

- Destruction of hepatocytes resulting in significant liver injury affecting the ability of the liver to perform its usual functions.
- Presenting symptoms and signs are related to hepatocellular dysfunction.
- Fulminant liver failure is acute liver disease complicated by encephalopathy within 8 weeks of onset of symptoms.

CAUSES

- See Figure 4.3.

CLINICAL FEATURES

- Presenting symptoms:
  - Nausea.
  - Anorexia.
  - Fatigue.
  - Confusion (hepatic encephalopathy):
    - Failure of the liver to remove nitrogenous compounds and toxins derived from the gut owing to loss of liver cell function.
    - These toxins cause impaired neural function through cytotoxicity, cell swelling and depletion of glutamine.
  - Coma (cerebral oedema).
- Examination:
  - Asterixis: flapping movements of the hand on wrist extension.
  - Jaundice.
  - Hepatosplenomegaly.
  - Signs of chronic liver disease (e.g. spider naevi).
  - Ascites:
    - Portal hypertension results in increased release of vasodilators (i.e. nitric oxide).
    - This leads to peripheral vasodilatation causing decreased blood pressure, and reduced renal blood flow, which activates the renin–angiotensin pathway.
    - This results in sodium and fluid retention.
  - Bleeding tendency:
    - Due to decreased synthesis of clotting factors and inhibitory proteins.
    - May manifest as bleeding gums, bruising or petechiae.

MANAGEMENT

- For immediate management, see Figure 4.3.
- Management of any precipitating cause.

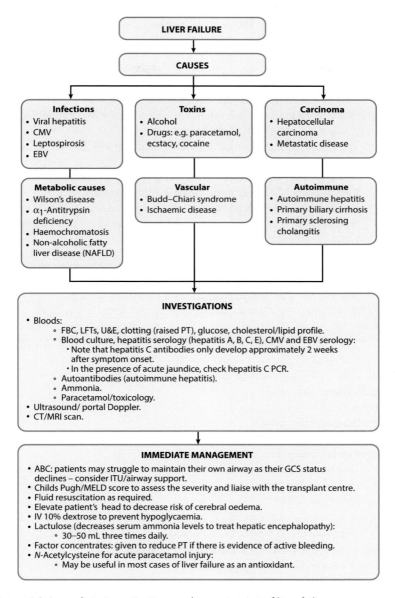

LIVER FAILURE

↓

CAUSES

Infections
- Viral hepatitis
- CMV
- Leptospirosis
- EBV

Toxins
- Alcohol
- Drugs: e.g. paracetamol, ecstacy, cocaine

Carcinoma
- Hepatocellular carcinoma
- Metastatic disease

Metabolic causes
- Wilson's disease
- α_1-Antitrypsin deficiency
- Haemochromatosis
- Non-alcoholic fatty liver disease (NAFLD)

Vascular
- Budd–Chiari syndrome
- Ischaemic disease

Autoimmune
- Autoimmune hepatitis
- Primary biliary cirrhosis
- Primary sclerosing cholangitis

INVESTIGATIONS
- Bloods:
  - FBC, LFTs, U&E, clotting (raised PT), glucose, cholesterol/lipid profile.
  - Blood culture, hepatitis serology (hepatitis A, B, C, E), CMV and EBV serology:
    - Note that hepatitis C antibodies only develop approximately 2 weeks after symptom onset.
    - In the presence of acute jaundice, check hepatitis C PCR.
  - Autoantibodies (autoimmune hepatitis).
  - Ammonia.
  - Paracetamol/toxicology.
- Ultrasound/ portal Doppler.
- CT/MRI scan.

↓

IMMEDIATE MANAGEMENT
- ABC: patients may struggle to maintain their own airway as their GCS status declines – consider ITU/airway support.
- Childs Pugh/MELD score to assess the severity and liaise with the transplant centre.
- Fluid resuscitation as required.
- Elevate patient's head to decrease risk of cerebral oedema.
- IV 10% dextrose to prevent hypoglycaemia.
- Lactulose (decreases serum ammonia levels to treat hepatic encephalopathy):
  - 30–50 mL three times daily.
- Factor concentrates: given to reduce PT if there is evidence of active bleeding.
- N-Acetylcysteine for acute paracetamol injury:
  - May be useful in most cases of liver failure as an antioxidant.

Figure 4.3 Immediate investigations and management of liver failure.

- Antibiotics given if there is any evidence of infection, or in the presence of a variceal haemorrhage:
  - Antifungals: up to 20% of patients may have systemic fungal infections.

- Correction of clotting if there is acute bleeding (factor concentrates, vitamin K).
- Management of ascites:
  - No added salt diet.
  - Pharmacological management: spironolactone, furosemide.
  - Abdominal paracentesis for large volume ascites.
- Liver transplantation is the gold standard treatment for liver failure which fails to respond to supportive measures:
  - The King's College Hospital criteria are used (see MICRO-reference box).
- Other options:
  - Auxiliary liver transplantation: donor graft implanted beside native liver to provide support until the native liver recovers.
  - Extracorporeal liver support: remove circulating toxins, but do not replace other liver functions (e.g. molecular adsorbent recirculation system [MARS]).

MICRO-reference

To review the King's College Hospital criteria for transplantation in liver failure, see: http://www.medicalcriteria.com/criteria/gas_liver_transp.htm

---

COMPLICATIONS

- Sepsis: bacterial/fungal.
- Ascites.
- Hepatic encephalopathy.
- Variceal bleeding.
- Hepatorenal syndrome:
  - Due to marked vasoconstriction of the renal arteries resulting in oliguria and sodium retention.
- Multiple organ failure.

PROGNOSIS

- Prognosis is dependent upon the underlying aetiology.
- Factors associated with poor prognosis:
  - Increasing age.
  - Drug-induced/hepatitis C-induced liver failure has worse prognosis.
  - Late-onset failure carries a worse prognosis than fulminant failure.
- Prognostic scoring systems:
  - Child-Pugh classification.
  - Model for End-Stage Liver Disease (MELD).
  - United Kingdom Model for End-Stage Liver Disease (UKELD).

4.3 ALCOHOL WITHDRAWAL

DEFINITION

- Constellation of symptoms occurring due to withdrawal from alcohol in a patient who has become physically dependent due to excessive consumption:
  - Current guidelines for maximum alcohol consumption are 21 units per week for males and 14 units per week for females.
  - Onset of symptoms is approximately 6–8 hours after their last drink.
  - Symptoms peak at 10–30 hours and subside after 2 days.
- The patient will have exhibited earlier features of alcohol dependence including:
  - Withdrawal symptoms.
  - Primacy: alcohol becomes most important in the patient's life.
  - Increasing tolerance.
  - Out of control drinking.
  - Unsuccessful attempts to cut down.
  - Disruption of everyday life: relationships, work, hobbies.
  - Continued use despite the knowledge it is causing harm.
- There are many clinical tools available for assessing a patient's risk of alcohol dependence (see MICRO-facts box) and for assessing alcohol withdrawal (the Clinical Institute Withdrawal Assessment for Alcohol Scale, Revised [CIWA-AR]):
  - The Fast Alcohol Screening Test (FAST) screening tool is often used in clinical practice as it can be completed relatively quickly.
  - The Alcohol Use Disorders Identification Test (AUDIT) questionnaire is also used as a screening tool.

MICRO-facts

FAST (Fast Alcohol Screening Test):

	SCORING SYSTEM				
	0	1	2	3	4
How often have you had 6 or more units (8 units if male) on a single occasion in the last year?	Never	Less than monthly	Monthly	Weekly	Daily/most days

continued...

continued...

	SCORING SYSTEM				
	0	1	2	3	4
How often during the last year have you failed to do what is normally expected from you because of drinking?	Never	Less than monthly	Monthly	Weekly	Daily/ most days
How often during the last year have you been unable to remember what happened the night before because of drinking?	Never	Less than monthly	Monthly	Weekly	Daily/ most days
Has a relative, friend, doctor or other health worker been concerned about your drinking/suggest you cut down?	No		Yes but not in the last year		Yes in the last year

A score of more than 3 indicates dangerous alcohol consumption.

MICRO-reference
For information on the AUDIT screening test for alcohol dependence, see: http://whqlibdoc.who.int/hq/2001/who_msd_msb_01.6a.pdf

CLINICAL FEATURES

- History:
  - Sweating.
  - Tremor.
  - Anxiety.
  - Nausea and vomiting.
  - Agitation.
- Examination:
  - Hypertension.
  - Tachycardia.
  - Dilated pupils.

COMPLICATIONS

- Delirium tremens:
  - Occurs in less than 5% of patients with withdrawal.
  - Generally occurs approximately 2–3 days following cessation of alcohol.
  - A severe state of withdrawal in which the patient may experience the following symptoms:
    - Tremor.
    - Fits (12–48 hours after cessation of drinking):
      - Usually generalized tonic–clonic seizures.
    - Hallucinations: may be visual, auditory or tactile.
    - Altered cognitive function:
      - Confusion.
      - Stupor.

MICRO-facts

Immediate management of delirium tremens:
- Keep patient comfortable, in a well lit room.
- Benzodiazepines (chlordiazepoxide or lorazepam):
  - Can be given as a loading dose followed by on demand.
- Antipsychotic medication (haloperidol, olanzapine).
- IV fluids and Pabrinex.

- Wernicke's encephalopathy:
  - Caused by deficiency of vitamin B_1 (thiamine).
  - Causes the classic triad of symptoms: ophthalmoplegia, global confusion, ataxia of trunk and lower limbs.
  - May progress to Korsakoff's syndrome if untreated:
    - Characterized by retrograde and anterograde amnesia.
    - Confabulation, lack of insight and minimal content in conversation.
    - Apathy.

MICRO-reference

For NICE clinical guidelines on diagnosis and management of alcohol-use disorders, visit: http://publications.nice.org.uk/alcohol-use-disorders-diagnosis-and-clinical-management-of-alcohol-related-physical-complications-cg100/guidance#wernickes-encephalopathy

Gastroenterology

ALCOHOL WITHDRAWAL

↓

IMMEDIATE MANAGEMENT
• Immediate hospital admission for patients in acute withdrawal.
• ABCDE and fluid resuscitation as required.
• Benzodiazepines:
    ◦ Chlordiazepoxide generally used.
    ◦ Given as a reducing regimen over 3–5 days.
    ◦ Use lorazepam if there is any evidence of advanced liver disease:
        • Has a shorter half-life.
        • Therefore less likely to accumulate, causing cognitive and respiratory depression.
• IV Pabrinex:
    ◦ Includes thiamine to decrease risk of developing Wernicke's encephalopathy.
• Beta-blockers.
• Carbamazepine (may be offered as an alternative to benzodiazepines).
• Antipsychotics:
    ◦ Used to treat hallucinations.

↓

FURTHER MANAGEMENT
• Nurse in a well-lit environment.
• Regular assessments of withdrawal/delirium tremens: e.g. CIWA score.
• Disulfiram:
    ◦ Produces unpleasant symptoms when patient consumes alcohol: nausea and vomiting, headache, sweating.
    ◦ Must not be given within 12 hours of acute alcohol withdrawal.
    ◦ May cause acute liver injury.
• Naltrexone:
    ◦ Reduces the positive psychological effects of alcohol experienced by the patient.
• Acamprosate:
    ◦ Increase likelihood of abstinence following withdrawal.
    ◦ Reduces craving for alcohol.
• All medications are to be used alongside psychological support:
    ◦ Group therapy (e.g. Alcoholics Anonymous).
    ◦ Management of any co-existing depression.

Figure 4.4 Management of alcohol withdrawal.

4.4 LIVER MASS

DEFINITION

- A discrete lesion within the liver, usually found on imaging during investigations for clinical symptoms, or on abnormal LFTs.

AETIOLOGY

- Benign lesions:
    - Polycystic liver disease.
    - Solitary cysts (congenital).

- Parasitic liver cysts: hydatid disease.
- Haemangioma.
- Liver abscess.
- Focal nodular hyperplasia (benign; may be mistaken for adenoma).
- Benign tumours: hepatocellular adenoma.
- Malignant tumours:
  - Hepatocellular carcinoma.
  - Intrahepatic cholangiocarcinoma.
  - Secondary lesions.

INVESTIGATIONS

- Blood tests:
  - LFTs: usually normal with liver cysts/haemangiomas/benign liver tumours.
  - Hydatid serology.
  - Alpha-fetoprotein:
    - May be raised in viral hepatitis or chronic liver disease.
    - Values >500 ng/mL are diagnostic of hepatocellular carcinoma.
  - CA 19-9: elevated in biliary and pancreatic malignancies.
- Imaging:
  - Ultrasound scan: differentiates between solid and cystic masses.
  - Multiphase CT.
  - Contrast MRI.
- Liver biopsy: biopsy of focal lesion.
- Laparoscopy.

MANAGEMENT

- Benign lesions often require no treatment once diagnosis confirmed.
- Liver abscesses require drainage and antibiotics and identification of the source of infection:
  - This is usually bowel (e.g. diverticulitis) or biliary tract (e.g. cholangitis).
- Hydatid cysts should be treated with albendazole/mebendazole and resected.
- Hepatic adenomas can rupture and can undergo malignant transformation so should be resected.
- For management of hepatocellular carcinoma, see Chapter 10.

Gastroenterology

4.5 ABNORMAL LIVER FUNCTION TESTS

DEFINITION

- Abnormal LFTs may be due to either primary problems within the liver, or may be a sign of disease elsewhere.

RISK FACTORS

- Chronic liver disease.
- NSAID use.
- Previous GI bleed.
- Upper GI malignancy.

AETIOLOGY

- Aminotransferases:
  - Includes alanine aminotransferase (ALT) and aspartate aminotransferase (AST).
  - ALT is a more specific marker of liver function than AST:
    - Increase in ALT is due to hepatocyte injury.
    - Very high levels seen in acute paracetamol overdose, acute ischaemic injury and acute viral hepatitis.
  - AST is also found in other tissues:
    - Increase in AST is seen in liver injury or muscle injury (e.g. following an MI, skeletal muscle disease, rhabdomyolysis).
- Bilirubin (see Section 4.1).
- Albumin:
  - Decreased albumin levels may indicate advanced liver disease:
    - Albumin has a half-life of 17–20 days and is therefore unaffected in the early stages of acute liver injury.
  - Low albumin may also be a sign of:
    - Nephrotic syndrome.
    - Protein-losing enteropathy.
    - Inflammation: albumin is a negative acute-phase protein.
- Gamma-glutamyl transferase (γGT):
  - Raised γGT may be a sign of cholestatic (obstructive) liver disease.
  - Alcohol and other hepatic enzyme-inducing substances (e.g. steroids, phenobarbitone) may cause elevated γGT.
- Alkaline phosphatase (ALP):
  - High levels of ALP may indicate cholestatic (obstructive liver disease) or liver infiltration (malignancy, granulomatous disease).

Table 4.1 **Table of LFT reference ranges (please note that different hospitals occasionally use different ranges so always check!)**

	NORMAL RANGE
Bilirubin	3–20 μmol/L
ALT	10–50 IU/L
ALP	30–150 IU/L
AST	10–50 IU/L
Albumin	30–50 g/L
γGT	<60 IU/L
Total protein	50–80 g/L

- ALP is also an isoenzyme of bone, and may become raised due to:
  - Osteomalacia/vitamin D deficiency.
  - Primary bone malignancy.
  - Bony metastasis.
  - Primary hyperparathyroidism.
  - Paget's disease.
  - Bone fracture.
  - Bone growth (children/teenagers).
- ALP is raised during late pregnancy:
  - Produced by the placenta.
- Prothrombin time (PT):
  - Prolonged in decompensated liver disease owing to reduced hepatic synthesis.
  - May also be prolonged in cholestatic disease.

MICRO-references
For further information on biopsy findings in patients with abnormal LFTs, see:
Skelly MM, James PD, Ryder SD. Findings on liver biopsy to investigate abnormal liver function tests in the absence of diagnostic serology. *Journal of Hepatology* 2001; 35(2): 195–199.
Paper available from: http://www.sciencedirect.com/science/article/pii/S0168827801000940#

Gastroenterology

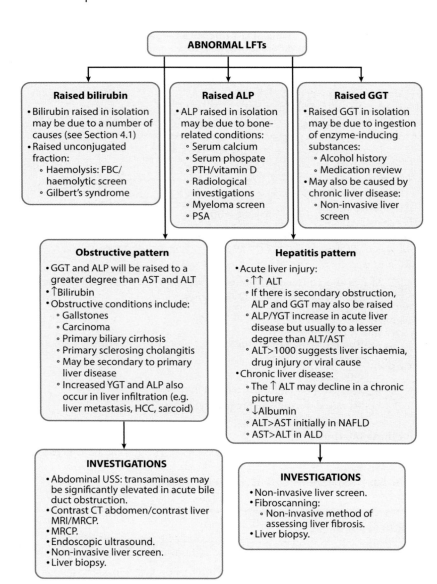

Figure 4.5 Interpretation of abnormal liver function tests.

MICRO-case

A 56-year-old overweight woman with jaundice is admitted onto the gastroenterology ward following a referral by her GP. The patient reports suffering intermittent abdominal pain over the preceding 2 months that has increased over the last week. She has lost a half stone in weight owing to reduced appetite. On examination, this pain is localized to the right hypochondrium. Blood tests, including FBC, U&E, LFTs, serum amylase and a clotting screen, are requested. The LFTs show the following abnormalities: bilirubin 52 μmol/L, ALT 78 IU/L, alkaline phosphatase 240 IU/L, γGT 290 IU/L, amylase 90 U/mL.

From these results, the doctor suspects that the patient is most likely suffering from gallstones and requests an abdominal ultrasound scan. This demonstrates multiple gallbladder stones and a slightly dilated common bile duct. Subsequently, however, the patient becomes pyrexial and tachycardic. Repeat bloods are taken including an FBC, CRP and blood cultures. The FBC reveals an elevated white cell count of 15×10^9/L.

Suspecting that the patient is now suffering from acute cholangitis, the doctor requests blood cultures, starts the patient on intravenous co-amoxiclav and organizes an MRCP which confirms two small stones in a 12-mm common bile duct. The patient is subsequently referred for urgent ERCP to remove her bile duct stones and allow biliary drainage.

Key points:

- When a patient presents with jaundice, a number of blood tests should be ordered in order to establish the underlying cause:
  - LFTs, FBC and clotting should initially be checked (can often help to differentiate between cholestatic and hepatic disorders).
  - A clotting screen should always be checked in case patients later require biliary intervention (e.g. ERCP, biopsy).
- Abdominal ultrasound is the investigation of choice for suspected gallstones, as the test has a high sensitivity.
- A diagnosis of gallstones may be complicated by acute cholangitis in approximately 9% of patients.
- Immediate management of cholangitis is with blood cultures to determine the causative agent, and antibiotics targeted to the underlying pathogen.
- Weight loss is common with symptomatic gallstone disease and does not necessarily suggest carcinoma of the pancreas. Pain is unusual in pancreatic cancer at diagnosis.

Gastroenterology

5 Oesophagus

5.1 ANATOMY

- A 25-cm-long hollow tube connecting the pharynx to the stomach.
- Functions as a transporter of ingested food in a delicately coordinated fashion.
- Histologically it comprises four concentric layers:
  - Mucosal layer (non-keratinized stratified squamous epithelium).
  - Submucosal layer.
  - Muscular layer.
  - External adventitia layer.
- It does not have any serosa.
- Muscle layer:
  - Consists of striated muscle in the proximal one-third and smooth muscle in the distal two-thirds.
  - Two sphincters control the ingested food material at both ends of the oesophagus:
    - The upper oesophageal sphincter (UOS) opens to let the food bolus in and rapidly closes afterwards to prevent aspiration.
    - The lower oesophageal sphincter (LOS) closes after food enters the stomach to prevent oesophageal reflux.
  - There are two muscle layers in the oesophagus:
    - The inner circular muscle fibres.
    - The outer longitudinal muscle fibres.
- Innervation:
  - Recurrent laryngeal branches of the vagus nerve supply the striated muscle of the proximal third.
  - Nerve supply to the smooth muscle of the lower two-thirds is also from the parasympathetic branches of the vagus nerve.
  - There are two parasympathetic plexuses located in the oesophageal wall:
    - Meissner ganglia (submucosal plexus) located in the submucosa.
    - Auerbach ganglia (myenteric plexus) located between the two muscular layers.
  - Sympathetic nerve branches from the 4th–6th thoracic spinal cord modify contraction amplitude, velocity and LOS tone (see Figure 5.1).

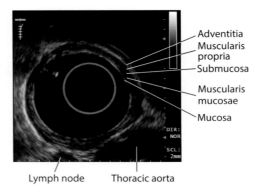

Figure 5.1 Endoscopic ultrasound image showing the anatomy of the oesophagus.

5.2 GASTRO-OESOPHAGEAL REFLUX DISEASE

DEFINITION

- Frequent retrograde flow of the gastroduodenal contents into the oesophagus.
- Causes a variety of symptoms and may result in damage to the oesophageal mucosa (and to lesser extent to the upper/lower respiratory system).

EPIDEMIOLOGY

- It is the most common digestive disease.
- The prevalence of the disease is increasing in Western countries.
- Incidence increases with age (especially after 40 years of age).
- Males and females are similarly affected.
- There is a direct association between body mass index and reflux symptoms.

PATHOPHYSIOLOGY

- An abnormality of the LOS plays a crucial role in gastro-oesophageal reflux disease (GORD) pathophysiology:
    - Hypotensive LOS.
    - Inappropriate transient lower oesophageal relaxation on a frequent basis.
    - Anatomical distortion (hiatus hernia) can directly affect LOS function.
- Gastric factors that increase risk of GORD:
    - Post-prandial over-expansion of the stomach.
    - Increased intra-abdominal pressure due to obesity.
    - Gastroparesis.
    - Increased gastric acid production (less frequent).

- Some medications can reduce LOS pressure and contribute to symptoms of GORD:
  - Oestrogens.
  - β-Adrenergic agonists.
  - Calcium channel blockers.
- Various foods and lifestyle behaviours can precipitate the disease:
  - Smoking.
  - Alcohol.
  - Caffeine.

CLINICAL FEATURES

- History:
  - Chest pain (retrosternal burning sensation that travels up to the neck).
  - Acid regurgitation.
  - Chronic cough.
  - Sore throat (pharyngitis).
- Red flag symptoms that necessitate urgent upper gastrointestinal (GI) evaluation:
  - Dysphagia.
  - Odynophagia.
  - Weight loss.
  - Upper GI bleeding.
  - Advanced age at presentation (55 or over).
  - Anaemia.
- Examination:
  - Hoarseness of voice.
  - Tracheal stenosis.
  - Halitosis.
  - Dental erosion.

INVESTIGATIONS

- A thorough history followed by a trial of PPI therapy is normally sufficient to diagnose the classical forms of GORD with no red flag symptoms.
- Further investigations:
  - Upper GI endoscopy.
  - Barium studies.
  - Ambulatory 24-hour pH and impedance studies.
  - Gastric emptying studies.

MANAGEMENT

- Lifestyle modification measures:
  - Smoking cessation.
  - Weight loss.

Gastroenterology

- Avoidance of late-night eating before going to sleep.
- Smaller and more frequent meals.
- Limiting certain foods in daily diet (e.g. caffeine, alcohol, fatty foods, carbonated drinks etc.).
- Pharmacological intervention:
  - Antacids.
  - H_2 receptor blockers.
  - PPIs.
  - Prokinetics.
- Surgical intervention:
  - May be offered to those who have failed maximum medical therapy or do not wish to continue long-term medication despite good medical response:
    - Anti-reflux surgery (e.g. Nissen fundoplication).
    - Endoscopic gastroplication (EndoCinch): suturing technique.
    - Endoscopic Stretta procedure: radio-ablation technique.

COMPLICATIONS

- Oesophageal stricture.
- Barrett's oesophagus (see Section 5.3).
- Adenocarcinoma.
- Extra-oesophageal complications:
  - Aspiration pneumonia.
  - Pulmonary fibrosis.
  - Asthma.
  - Chronic cough.

5.3 BARRETT'S OESOPHAGUS

DEFINITION

- Replacement of the normal squamous epithelium with specialized columnar epithelium with evidence of intestinal metaplasia (goblet cells).
- Salmon coloured mucosa starting from the gastro-oesophageal junction (GOJ) and extending proximally to various lengths.
- The presence of such metaplastic changes is the strongest risk factor for development of oesophageal carcinoma.

EPIDEMIOLOGY

- 6–12% of patients undergoing endoscopy for symptomatic reflux are discovered to have developed Barrett's oesophagus.
- 1–2% of unselected patients undergoing endoscopy are discovered to have the condition.

RISK FACTORS

- GORD: exposes the distal oesophagus to acid and bile salts.
- Hiatus hernia.
- Weak LOS tone.
- Decreased amplitude of distal oesophageal peristalsis (reduced acid clearance).
- Male sex.
- Advanced age.
- Caucasian ethnicity.
- Smoking.
- Heavy alcohol use.

INVESTIGATIONS

- Initial investigation:
    - Upper GI endoscopy coupled with histological confirmation is the gold standard investigation.
    - The use of high-resolution endoscopes is recommended.
- Surveillance:
    - The British Society of Gastroenterology (BSG) advises surveillance with upper GI endoscopy:
        - Segments less than 3 cm – every 3–5 years.
        - Segments of 3 cm or more – every 2–3 years.
    - 6-monthly OGD is recommended if low-grade dysplasia is found.

MANAGEMENT

- Lifestyle modification (as for GORD).
- Pharmacological intervention:
    - Lifelong PPI therapy should be advised to every patient with a diagnosis of Barrett's oesophagus with GORD symptoms.
- Surgical intervention:
    - In cases of confirmed high-grade dysplasia or intramucosal cancer, a multidisciplinary team decision should be made for consideration of endoscopic resection followed by radiofrequency ablative therapy or surgery.

COMPLICATIONS

- Adenocarcinoma:
    - Incidence of 0.2–0.4% per year.
    - Intestinal metaplasia → low-grade dysplasia → high-grade dysplasia → adenocarcinoma.
    - Direct association between the length of Barrett's mucosa segment and the risk of adenocarcinoma.

Gastroenterology

> **MICRO-reference**
> Bennett C, Vakil N, Bergman J, et al. Consensus Statements for
> Management of Barrett's Dysplasia and Early-Stage Esophageal
> Adenocarcinoma, based on a Delphi process. *Gastroenterology* 2012;
> 143(2): 336–346. See: http://www.gastrojournal.org/article/S0016-
> 5085(12)00614-2/fulltext

5.4 HIATUS HERNIA

DEFINITION

- Prolapse of a portion of the stomach through the diaphragmatic oesophageal hiatus.
- Classified into sliding or rolling hiatus hernia (see Figure 5.2):
  - Sliding:
    - The part of stomach immediately below the GOJ prolapses through the oesophageal hiatus into the chest cavity.
  - Rolling (para-oesophageal):
    - The cardia or fundus of the stomach herniates upwards into the chest cavity, alongside the oesophagus through the diaphragmatic hiatus while leaving the GOJ within the abdominal cavity.
  - Mixed:
    - Combination of the above.

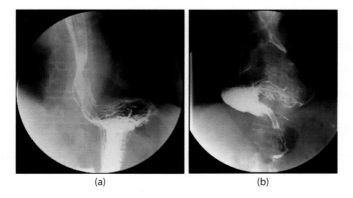

(a) (b)

Figure 5.2 Barium swallow images. (a) A simple sliding hiatus hernia and (b) a more complex para-oesophageal hiatus hernia. Note the dual chamber cardiac pace-maker also *in situ*.

Gastroenterology

RISK FACTORS

- Pregnancy.
- Obesity.
- Large volume ascites.
- Age related loss of elasticity and muscle weakening.
- Female gender.
- Constipation.

CLINICAL FEATURES

- History:
  - Generally asymptomatic.
  - Sliding hiatus hernia:
    - Can present with symptoms of GORD (see Section 5.2).
  - Rolling hiatus hernia:
    - Substernal fullness/pain.
    - Nausea.
    - Dysphagia.
    - Acute abdominal pain if complicated by gastric volvulus.

INVESTIGATIONS

- Barium swallow:
  - Modality of choice.
  - Can differentiate between the two types of hernia with high accuracy.
- OGD:
  - Used to investigate complications such as GORD, Barrett's oesophagus, ulcer or tumour.
- CXR:
  - May reveal a large hiatus hernia.

MANAGEMENT

- Pharmacological intervention:
  - GORD management (see Section 5.2).
- Surgical intervention:
  - Indicated in cases where there are severe complications associated with GORD, or for complications of para-oesophageal hiatus hernia (strangulation, volvulus).
  - Common surgical techniques include:
    - Nissen fundoplication.
    - Belsey fundoplication.
    - Hill repair.

Gastroenterology

COMPLICATIONS

- Increased risk of GORD.
- Oesophagitis.
- Erosions at the diaphragmatic hiatus (Cameron ulcers).
- Discrete oesophageal ulcers leading to iron deficiency anaemia.
- Gastric volvulus and incarceration of the hiatus hernia (only with rolling hiatus hernia).

5.5 ACHALASIA

DEFINITION

- The literal meaning is 'failure to relax'.
- Neuropathic motor disorder of the oesophageal smooth muscle:
  - LOS fails to relax in response to swallowing and the oesophageal body loses its normal peristalsis.

EPIDEMIOLOGY

- Incidence is about 0.5–1.5 per 100,000.
- Usually occurs in the third to fifth decades.

PATHOPHYSIOLOGY

- Decreased number of intramural non-cholinergic non-adrenergic myenteric ganglion cells due to unknown cause.
- Cholinergic neurons can also be affected in advanced disease.

AETIOLOGY

- Primary idiopathic achalasia is the most common form of the disease in Western countries.
- Chagas disease:
  - An infection due to *Trypanosoma cruzi*.
  - Initiates an immunological attack against the ganglion cells of the oesophagus.
- Secondary achalasia may be caused by:
  - Varicella zoster infection.
  - Tumours infiltrating the lower oesophagus.
  - Paraneoplastic syndrome (due to small cell lung cancer).
  - Lymphoma.
  - Neurodegenerative disorders.

CLINICAL FEATURES

- History:
  - Dysphagia:
    - Commonly both liquids and solids.
    - Typically fluctuates.
  - Regurgitation.
  - Chest pain.
  - Weight loss.
  - Cough.

INVESTIGATIONS

- Chest X-ray:
  - A fluid level may be seen in the oesophagus and characteristically there is an absence of the gastric air bubble.
- Barium swallow:
  - Shows oesophageal dilatation.
  - The classic fluoroscopy picture is the 'bird's beak' appearance with loss of normal peristalsis in the distal two-thirds of the oesophagus.
- OGD:
  - Helpful in ruling out secondary causes of achalasia such as cancer.
- Manometry:
  - Shows low-amplitude, non-propagating contractions with failure of the LOS to relax on swallowing.

MANAGEMENT

- Pharmacological intervention (usually shows only short-term efficacy):
  - Nifedipine.
  - Sublingual isosorbide dinitrate.
  - Sublingual nitroglycerine.
  - Sildenafil.
- Endoscopic intervention:
  - Endoscopic injection of botulinum toxin into the LOS:
    - Short-term effect with symptom recurrence after 6–12 months requiring further injection.
  - Endoscopic balloon dilatation of the LOS:
    - Approximately 90% respond at 1 year, but approximately a third of patients require repeat dilatations.
- Surgical myotomy:
  - Open or laparoscopic.

- Oesophagectomy:
  - Only in rare, extreme and refractory cases which fail to respond to the above treatments.

COMPLICATIONS

- Squamous cell carcinoma (16-fold increased risk).
- Oesophageal fibrosis due to repeated botulinum toxin injections.
- GORD symptoms following surgical myotomy and to a lesser degree following endoscopic pneumatic dilatation.

5.6 OESOPHAGEAL SPASM

DEFINITION

- Motility disorder of the oesophagus typically split into two categories (see Figure 5.3):
  - Hypermotility (spastic) disorders:
    - Diffuse oesophageal spasm (uncoordinated, non-peristaltic contractions).
    - Hypertensive peristalsis (nutcracker oesophagus).
  - Hypomotility disorders:
    - Scleroderma (failure of muscle contraction, incompetent LOS).
    - Idiopathic hypomotility.

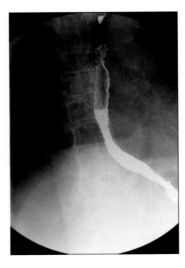

Figure 5.3 Barium swallow showing oesophageal spasm.

Gastroenterology

CLINICAL FEATURES

- History:
  - Substernal chest pain and odynophagia (usually with hypermotility subtypes).
  - Heartburn (usually with hypomotility subtypes).
  - Intermittent dysphagia to both solid and liquid.
  - Regurgitation.
  - Globus hystericus.

INVESTIGATIONS

- Barium swallow:
  - Shows numerous simultaneous contractions.
  - Non-propulsive oesophageal contractions.
- Manometry:
  - Helpful for diagnosis as well as exclusion of achalasia.
- OGD can help in excluding alternative diagnoses such as:
  - Oesophageal stricture.
  - Malignancy.
  - Hiatus hernia.
  - Eosinophilic oesophagitis.
  - Reflux disease.

MANAGEMENT

- Pharmacological intervention (minimally effective in most cases):
  - Calcium channel blockers.
  - Nitrates.
  - Tricyclic antidepressants.
  - Sildenafil.
- Endoscopic intervention:
  - Endoscopic botulinum toxin injection just above the LOS may improve the symptoms in some patients temporarily.

MICRO-print

Eosinophilic oesophagitis is an uncommon cause of dysphagia, and less commonly heartburn, that does not respond to PPI therapy. The diagnosis is made based on clinical presentation alongside the histopathological finding of high tissue eosinophils after excluding other disorders with similar clinicopathological features, especially GORD and primary eosinophilic gastroenteritis. It is often associated with atopy and is usually treated by use of swallowed inhaled corticosteroids. Exclusion diets to identify precipitating foods can be successful in some patients.

Gastroenterology

- Endoscopic balloon dilatation of the LOS can be considered in patients with refractory dysphagic symptoms with variable success.
- Surgical intervention:
  - In extreme cases not responsive to medical and endoscopic treatments, surgical myotomy followed by anti-reflux surgery is an option.

5.7 OESOPHAGEAL CANCER

PATHOPHYSIOLOGY

- Primary malignancies are the most common tumours of the oesophagus:
  - Adenocarcinoma and squamous cell carcinoma are the most common forms, accounting for 90% of malignancies.
  - Other malignancies include small cell carcinoma, melanoma, sarcoma, lymphoma and metastatic carcinoma.

EPIDEMIOLOGY

- Oesophageal cancer affects more than 450,000 people worldwide.
- It is the ninth most common cancer in the UK with an incidence of 13.6:100,000.
- Squamous cell carcinoma is the most common oesophageal cancer worldwide.
- In the UK, USA, Australia and some Western European countries, the incidence of adenocarcinoma is now higher than that of squamous cell carcinoma.

RISK FACTORS

- Squamous cell carcinoma:
  - Tobacco.
  - Alcohol.
  - Drinking very hot beverages.
  - Plummer–Vinson syndrome: a condition characterized by formation of oesophageal webs, progressive dysphagia and iron deficiency anaemia.
  - Tylosis: congenital hyperkeratosis of palms of the hands and soles of the feet.
  - Nutritional deficiencies (vitamin C).
  - Poor oral hygiene.
  - Achalasia.
  - History of previous thoracic radiation.

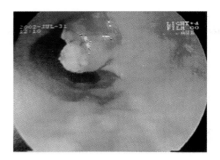

Figure 5.4 Endoscopic image of oesophageal carcinoma.

- Adenocarcinoma:
  - Barrett's oesophagus is the strongest risk factor for oesophageal adenocarcinoma.
  - Other risk factors:
    - Obesity.
    - Male sex.
    - Increased age.
    - Low fibre diet.
    - History of thoracic radiation.
    - Tobacco use.
    - GORD.

CLINICAL FEATURES

- History:
  - Dysphagia:
    - Begins with solids and progresses to liquids in a short period.
  - Odynophagia (painful swallowing):
    - Pain may radiate to the central chest or back.
- Examination:
  - Weight loss.
  - Hoarseness of voice.
  - Lymphadenopathy.

INVESTIGATIONS

- Barium swallow.
- OGD: tissue biopsy for confirmation of diagnosis.
- CT staging:
  - Chest, abdomen and pelvis.
  - Required to screen for distant metastasis.

Gastroenterology

- PET scanning:
  - Required in patients who are potential surgical candidates if there is no evidence of distant metastasis on CT staging.
- Endoscopic ultrasound:
  - Very useful if no metastatic disease is found for accurate regional staging with TNM (tumour, nodes, metastases) classification.

MICRO-reference

Visit the National Cancer Institute online for the full TNM staging of gastric cancer: http://www.cancer.gov/cancertopics/pdq/treatment/gastric/HealthProfessional/page3

MANAGEMENT

- A multidisciplinary approach to every individual is of utmost importance taking into account the patient's performance status, medical comorbidities and wishes in directing the best treatment.
- Treatment options are very variable depending on:
  - The stage of the disease.
  - The patient's performance status.
  - Comorbid conditions.
  - Personal wishes.
- Treatment options include:
  - Early disease localized to mucosa:
    - Endoscopic mucosal resection (EMR)/radiofrequency ablation.
  - Resectable disease:
    - Neoadjuvant chemotherapy (commonly 5-fluorouracil and cisplatin) followed by oesophagectomy.
  - Palliative therapy:
    - Mechanical (stenting).
    - Radiotherapy.
    - Palliative chemotherapy.

PROGNOSIS

- The overall 5-year survival ranges from 5% to 25%, depending on the stage of the disease at diagnosis.
- Only 20–30% of all cases are suitable for surgical resection.
- Approximately 20–40% of cases undergoing surgery survive 3 years or more.
- 5-year survival for patients with high-grade dysplasia or T1 disease is 90%.

MICRO-facts

The UK Department of Health (DoH) recommends urgent referral for upper GI investigation in any patients with the following red flag symptoms:

- Dysphagia
- Odynophagia
- Weight loss
- Upper GI bleeding
- Anaemia
- Persistent new-onset dyspepsia (aged 55 or over)

The British Society of Gastroenterology (BSG) also recommends consideration of upper GI endoscopy for patients in any age group with clinical suspicion of malignancy even in the absence of alarm symptoms, as early localized tumours may not initially present with the above typical symptoms.

MICRO-case

A 56-year-old shopkeeper visits her GP with a 6-month history of worsening heartburn, intermittent water brash and epigastric pain (that occurs around an hour post-prandially, especially at nighttime). She has also noticed an early morning dry cough and slight hoarseness recently. She is overweight and is a smoker of 20 pack-years. Her GP previously advised her on lifestyle modifications including weight loss, smaller but more frequent meals, smoking cessation, minimizing alcohol consumption and at least a 3-hour gap between her last meal and sleeping. She has been on omeprazole 20 mg once a day for the past 2 years with an initial good response but recent relapse. She had been tested negative for *Helicobacter pylori* prior to this therapy. During the consultation she denies difficult or painful swallowing and recent weight loss. Her only regular medication is omeprazole.

On examination, her BMI is 33 and general examination is unremarkable.

Her GP makes an urgent referral for gastroscopy and also arranges for a CXR and FBC. Her gastroscopy shows moderate oesophagitis and a 4-cm hiatus hernia. The CXR is clear and her FBC is normal.

She is diagnosed with GORD. Special emphasis is placed on lifestyle modifications and her omeprazole is doubled to 20 mg twice a day taken half an hour before food with consideration to add ranitidine 150 mg at night. She responds well to the new regime.

continued...

Gastroenterology

continued...

Key points:

- Urgent gastroscopy should be considered for patients over 55 years of age with unexplained and persistent recent-onset dyspepsia alone as per NICE guidelines.
- PPI timing should be emphasized regarding taking the medication at least half an hour to an hour before food to be effective.
- Offer a PPI at the lowest dose possible to control the symptoms if long-term maintenance PPI therapy is required.
- If hoarseness does not improve with PPI, then ENT referral needs to be considered.
- The importance of lifestyle management should be explained; adequate weight loss usually prevents the need for long-term PPI.

6 Stomach and duodenum

6.1 ANATOMY

- The stomach can be divided into the following anatomical regions:
  - Cardia.
  - Fundus.
  - Body.
  - Antrum.
  - Pylorus.
- The gastric wall is made up of four layers:
  - Serosa.
  - Muscularis propria.
  - Submucosa.
  - Mucosa: lined with columnar epithelium.
- The muscularis propria comprises three muscle layers:
  - Outer longitudinal muscle.
  - Middle circular muscle.
  - Inner oblique muscle.
- The stomach is separated from the oesophagus by the lower oesophageal sphincter and the duodenum by the pyloric sphincter.

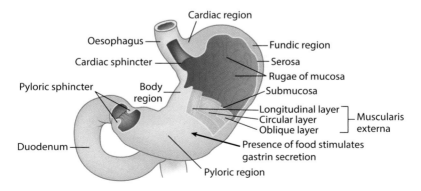

Figure 6.1 Anatomy of the stomach.

6.2 PHYSIOLOGY

- The cells lining the stomach produce many different secretions.
- These secretions produce a wide variety of effects and are strictly controlled by a number of different mechanisms (see Table 6.1).

6.3 PEPTIC ULCER DISEASE

DEFINITION

- Peptic ulcer disease encompasses both gastric and duodenal ulcers.
- A peptic ulcer is a break in the mucosal lining of the stomach or duodenum that extends through the muscularis mucosae and into the submucosa.
- More superficial breaks in the mucosa are termed 'erosions'.

EPIDEMIOLOGY

- More common in men than women (2:1).
- More common with increasing age.
- Duodenal ulcers are three times more common than gastric ulcers.
- Poor socioeconomic status is associated with increased risk of peptic ulcers.

AETIOLOGY/RISK FACTORS

- *Helicobacter pylori* infection:
  - This is a gram-negative, spiral or curved rod with flagellae.
  - It colonizes gastric mucosa causing underlying inflammation.
  - The organism survives by neutralizing the acidic environment of the stomach by converting urea to ammonia.
  - *H. pylori* is associated with duodenal ulcers in 95% of cases compared to 60–70% of gastric ulcers.
- Drugs:
  - NSAIDs.
  - Oral steroids (e.g. prednisolone).
  - Chemotherapy (e.g. 5-fluorouracil).
  - Cocaine.
  - Bisphosphonates.
- Alcohol abuse.
- Smoking.
- Stressful lifestyle.
- Hyperacidity: Zollinger–Ellison syndrome.
- Acute stress: surgery, trauma.

Gastroenterology

Table 6.1 **Physiology of stomach secretions**

	CELL OF ORIGIN	ACTION	STIMULATING FACTORS	INHIBITORY FACTORS
Hydrochloric acid (HCl)	Parietal cell (gastric fundus/body)	Activation of enzymes Inhibition of bacterial colonization	Gastrin Acetylcholine Histamine	Somatostatin
Intrinsic factor	Parietal cell	Facilitates B_{12} absorption in the terminal ileum		
Pepsinogen	Chief cell (gastric fundus/body)	Activated to pepsin by HCl Digestion of proteins/peptides	Activated by HCl Parasympathetic stimulation	
Gastrin	G cell (gastric antrum)	Controls gastric motility and secretion of HCl	Parasympathetic nervous system Presence of amino acids	Somatostatin Presence of HCl
Somatostatin	Enterochromaffin-like (ECL) cell (gastric fundus/body)	Regulation of gastric acid secretion	Presence of HCl	Parasympathetic nervous system
Histamine	ECL cell	Stimulates secretion of HCl		
Mucus	Mucous cell (throughout the stomach)	Forms a bicarbonate-rich protective layer around the stomach	Prostaglandins	

PATHOPHYSIOLOGY

- Breakdown of the mucosa occurs when there is an imbalance between the protective mechanisms of the stomach and the acidic nature of its contents:
  - Interruption of the mucus bicarbonate barrier lining the stomach:
    - *H. pylori* infection: secretes proteases that break down the protective mucus layer.
    - Reflux gastritis: reflux of bile into the stomach removes the mucus layer.
  - Damage to the epithelium:
    - Use of NSAIDs: prevents the production of prostaglandins:
      ○ Damage may be minimized by using enteric-coated preparations.
    - *H. pylori* infection: produces proteases and ammonia, which are toxic to the epithelium.
  - Acid hypersecretion, associated with duodenal ulceration:
    - *H. pylori* infection of the gastric antrum: results in increased gastrin production, stimulating acid secretion.
    - Zollinger–Ellison syndrome: gastrin-secreting tumours stimulate excessive acid secretion.
    - *H. pylori* infection of the gastric body is associated with gastric atrophy, reduced acid secretion and an increased risk of gastric ulcer due to direct toxic mechanism and an increased risk of gastric malignancy.

CLINICAL FEATURES

- Abdominal pain/dyspepsia:
  - Generally epigastric – may be described as 'burning'.
  - Typically relieved by food with duodenal ulcers.
  - Precipitated by food with gastric ulcers.
  - Radiating to the back: this may be a sign of a posterior ulcer.
- Nausea and vomiting.
- Symptoms related to bleeding:
  - Melaena.
  - Haematemesis/coffee-ground vomit.

MICRO-facts

In minor GI bleeds, the iron within the haeme molecules of the red blood cells becomes oxidized by the gastric acid; the resultant vomitus takes on a dark coffee-ground appearance. As a sign, coffee-ground vomiting should be interpreted by an experienced health professional, as any dark vomitus tends to be wrongly labelled as coffee-ground. Dip-stick testing of the vomitus should never be done as it is almost always positive, even in the absence of GI bleeding.

Gastroenterology

INVESTIGATIONS

- FBC:
    - Microcytic anaemia due to iron deficiency from chronic bleeding.
    - Normocytic anaemia in acute bleeding.
- Test for *H. pylori*:
    - Faecal antigen test.
    - Urea breath test:
        - Patient is asked to swallow a solution containing labelled urea.
        - The urease produced by *H. pylori* converts the urea to CO_2.
        - The test measures the exhalation of a labelled isotope of CO_2.
- Endoscopy and biopsy:
    - Used for the investigation and management of upper GI bleeding.
    - Used to exclude gastric cancer in the presence of alarm symptoms (see Chapter 3).

MICRO-facts

Before testing for *H. pylori* infection, the patient must have been taken off PPI medication for 2 weeks and antibiotic therapy for 4 weeks.

MANAGEMENT

- Treatment or withdrawal of the underlying cause:
    - *H. pylori* eradication therapy (see MICRO-facts box).
    - Stop NSAIDs and other causative drugs.
    - Decrease/stop alcohol.
    - Smoking cessation.
- Pharmacological intervention:
    - Proton pump inhibitor (PPI).
    - H_2 receptor antagonist.
- Endoscopic therapy – used in bleeding ulcers:
    - Injection of epinephrine.
    - Thermal coagulation.
    - Mechanical clipping.
    - Haemospray (inorganic adsorptive powder that is sprayed onto actively bleeding ulcers producing a stable mechanical plug).

Gastroenterology

> ## MICRO-facts
>
> Triple therapy for *H. pylori* eradication requires 7 days of the following:
>
> - One proton pump inhibitor:
>   - E.g. omeprazole 20 mg b.d.
> - Two antibiotics:
>   - E.g. clarithromycin 500 mg b.d.
>   - And amoxicillin 1 g b.d. or metronidazole 400 mg b.d.

COMPLICATIONS

- Haemorrhage:
  - Due to erosion of the ulcer into a vessel.
  - The Glasgow-Blatchford Bleeding Score may be used to assess the severity of upper GI bleeding and help to determine the management (see MICRO-reference box).
- Perforation:
  - More common in duodenal ulcers.
  - Risk of peritonitis.
- Obstruction:
  - May occur with ulcers in the pylorus, antrum or duodenum.

> ### MICRO-reference
> For more information on calculating the Glasgow-Blatchford Bleeding Score, see: http://www.mdcalc.com/glasgow-blatchford-bleeding-score-gbs/

6.4 GASTRITIS

DEFINITION

- Acute gastritis: acute inflammation of the stomach lining.
- Chronic gastritis: chronic inflammation of the stomach lining lasting months to years.

AETIOLOGY

- *H. pylori* infection.
- Smoking.
- Caffeine.
- Drugs – similar to those for peptic ulcer disease (see Section 6.3).
- Alcohol abuse: acute gastritis due to chemical injury.

- Autoimmune chronic gastritis (see Section 6.5):
  - Patients form antibodies against intrinsic factor and the parietal cells of the stomach.
  - This may result in a deficiency of B_{12} with associated achlorhydria.
- Reflux gastritis: caused by reflux of duodenal contents back into the stomach.
- Granulomatous causes: sarcoidosis, Crohn's disease.
- Hypertrophic gastritis:
  - Ménétrier's disease (rare premalignant disorder of the stomach characterized by giant gastric folds associated with epithelial hyperplasia).
- Lymphocytic gastritis: associated with coeliac disease.
- Eosinophilic gastritis:
  - Associated with peripheral eosinophilia and eosinophilic infiltration of various sites of the gastrointestinal tract.
  - May cause pain, vomiting, diarrhoea and anaemia.
- Acute stress.
- Portal hypertensive gastritis (associated with portal hypertension).

PATHOPHYSIOLOGY

- Injury to the mucosa of the stomach causes an inflammatory response with infiltration of neutrophils into the mucosal lining.
- Multiple erosions penetrate the superficial mucosa.
- The erosions may cause haemorrhage which leads to acute blood loss.

CLINICAL FEATURES

- History:
  - Nausea.
  - Vomiting.
  - Dyspepsia.
  - Haemorrhagic symptoms: coffee-ground haematemesis, melaena.
- Examination:
  - Epigastric pain: may be exacerbated by eating.

INVESTIGATIONS

- Test for *H. pylori* (see Section 6.3).
- FBC: to check for anaemia from blood loss.
- Test for serum B_{12}:
  - If this is low, test for serum anti-intrinsic factor and parietal cell antibodies.
- Upper GI endoscopy ± biopsy:
  - Urease test for *H. pylori*.
  - Histology for *H. pylori*/malignancy to exclude rare forms such as lymphocytic/eosinophilic gastritis.

Gastroenterology

MANAGEMENT

- Management of risk factors:
  - Withdrawal of NSAIDs or other damaging agents.
  - Reduced alcohol intake.
  - *H. pylori* eradication therapy if indicated (see Section 6.3):
    - If symptoms do not resolve after eradication, consider long-term acid suppression.
- Pharmacological therapy:
  - Antacids for symptomatic relief.
  - PPI or H_2 receptor antagonist: generally prescribed for 1 month.
  - Sucralfate: may act by protecting the gastric mucosa from acid/pepsin attack.

COMPLICATIONS

- If left untreated, the erosions may progress to form ulcers.
- Gastric carcinoma (see Section 6.7 for pathophysiology).
- MALT (mucosa-associated lymphoid tissue) lymphoma.
- Gastric non-Hodgkin's lymphoma: patients are six times more likely to be infected with *H. pylori*.

PROGNOSIS

- With treatment/withdrawal of the underlying cause, patients generally make a full recovery.

6.5 PERNICIOUS ANAEMIA

DEFINITION

- Autoimmune condition characterized by loss of parietal cells and subsequent failure of intrinsic factor production leading to a lack of vitamin B_{12} absorption.
- A megaloblastic, macrocytic anaemia secondary to vitamin B_{12} deficiency.

EPIDEMIOLOGY

- Affects 0.1% of the general population and 1.9% of those above 60 years of age.
- More common in females than males: 1.6:1.

RISK FACTORS

- Risk factors:
  - Other autoimmune disorders:
    - Addison's disease.
    - Type 1 diabetes mellitus.
    - Autoimmune thyroid disease.

- – Vitiligo.
- – Hypoparathyroidism.
- Family history.
- Associated factors:
  - Blood group A.
  - Blue eyes.
  - Fair hair.
  - Premature greying of hair.

PATHOPHYSIOLOGY

- Autoimmune destruction of parietal cells and chief cells:
  - Parietal cells produce hydrochloric acid and intrinsic factor.
  - Destruction therefore causes hypochlorhydria and a lack of intrinsic factor.
- All vitamin B_{12} comes from the diet: there is no endogenous production.
- Intrinsic factor is required for vitamin B_{12} absorption:
  - Binds to B_{12} in the stomach.
  - Absorbed in the terminal ileum (TI).
- Antibodies to parietal cells found in 90% of sufferers.
- Antibodies to intrinsic factor found in 50%.
- Other causes of B_{12} deficiency:
  - Total/partial gastrectomy.
  - Terminal ileal resection.
  - Intestinal disease affecting the TI (such as Crohn's disease).
  - Small bowel bacterial overgrowth.
  - Vegetarianism/veganism.
  - Chronic pancreatitis.
  - Fish tape worm infections.
- Vitamin B_{12} is required for DNA synthesis:
  - Defective DNA synthesis during production of red blood cells results in the production of large, fragile megaloblastic erythrocytes.
  - Rarely there is co-existing pancytopenia.

CLINICAL FEATURES

- Progressive onset of symptoms since liver stores of vitamin B_{12} last for several years.
- History:
  - Symptoms of anaemia: fatigue, dyspnoea, pre-syncope.
  - Weight loss.
  - Neurological symptoms:
    - – Paraesthesia in the hands and feet due to peripheral neuropathy.
    - – Gait ataxia/leg weakness.
    - – Dementia.

- Examination:
  - Pallor.
  - Mild jaundice secondary to increased red cell breakdown.
  - Glossitis (swollen tongue).
  - Angular stomatitis (fissuring of the corners of the mouth).
  - Neurological signs: optic atrophy, peripheral neuropathy, loss of joint position sense and vibration with a spastic paraparesis (subacute degeneration of the cord).

INVESTIGATIONS

- Serum vitamin B_{12}: low.
- FBC:
  - Low haemoglobin.
  - High MCV (mean corpuscular volume).
  - White cell count and platelets can be low in severe disease.
- Serum bilirubin: may be high due to increased red blood cell breakdown.
- Antibodies:
  - Parietal cell antibodies.
  - Intrinsic factor antibodies.
- Screening for other autoimmune conditions:
  - Thyroid function test (TFT).
  - Thyroid antibodies if indicated by the results of TFT.
  - Short Synacthen test.
  - Parathyroid hormone.
- Schilling test:
  - Differentiates pernicious anaemia from other megaloblastic anaemias.
  - Rarely used.

MICRO-facts

The Schilling test is used to differentiate between B_{12} deficiency due to a lack of intrinsic factor (pernicious anaemia) and malabsorption of B_{12} due to other causes.

Radioactive B_{12} is administered both with and without intrinsic factor and absorption is measured through measuring urinary excretion of B_{12} over 24 hours. If intrinsic factor increases absorption, then a lack of intrinsic factor is likely to be causative. If there is no difference in absorption, then the deficiency is likely due to another mechanism.

MANAGEMENT

- Pharmacological intervention:
  - Intramuscular vitamin B_{12} injections (hydroxocobalamin).

- For patients with co-existing folate deficiency:
  - Treat with vitamin B$_{12}$ first.
  - Treatment with folic acid can initially precipitate neurological complications.

COMPLICATIONS

- Increased risk of gastric cancer: around three times higher than in the general population.
- Neurological complications (see Section 6.5).

6.6 GASTROPARESIS

DEFINITION

- Reduced activity of the muscular wall of the stomach resulting in slow passage of stomach contents.
- Also called delayed gastric emptying.

AETIOLOGY

- Diabetes:
  - Autonomic damage to vagus nerve decreases stimulation of the stomach.
  - 30–60% of diabetic patients have a degree of gastroparesis.
- Partial gastrectomy.
- Systemic sclerosis.
- Anticholinergic medication:
  - Parkinson's disease medication.
  - Antipsychotics.
  - Antidepressants – predominately tricyclic antidepressants (TCAs).
  - Buscopan.
- Neurological cause: Parkinson's disease, spinal cord injury, myasthenia gravis.
- Hypothyroidism.
- Iatrogenic: post-surgery secondary to damage to vagus nerve.

PATHOPHYSIOLOGY

- The normal physiology of gastric emptying, largely under the control of the vagus, is grossly disturbed resulting in:
  - Increase in antral arrhythmias causing increase in antral pressure.
  - Poor antral expulsion and reduced gastric output.
  - Smooth muscle degeneration and fibrosis.
  - Depletion of the gastric pacemaker cells (interstitial Cajal cells).
  - Emptying of solids affected more than emptying of liquids.

CLINICAL FEATURES

- History:
  - Nausea and vomiting.
  - Early satiety.
  - Weight loss.
  - Lack of appetite.
  - Symptoms of gastro-oesophageal reflux.
- Examination:
  - Abdominal distension.

INVESTIGATIONS

- Oesophago-gastro-duodenoscopy (OGD):
  - Upper GI endoscopy.
  - To exclude other pathology.
- Gastric emptying study:
  - Radioactive isotope added to meal.
  - Scanner placed over abdomen to monitor gastric emptying.
- Ultrasound scan:
  - Can show antral and duodenal contractions as well as transpyloric flow.
- Electrogastrography (EGG):
  - Produces a graphical representation of the electrical activity of the stomach; measured fasting and after a test meal.
- Antroduodenal manometry: invasive procedure.

DIFFERENTIAL DIAGNOSIS

- Gastric outflow obstruction: e.g. tumour or peptic ulcer.

MANAGEMENT

- Lifestyle modifications:
  - Small, regular meals.
  - Liquid or puréed meals – liquid phase unaffected.
  - Low-fat and -fibre diet.
- Pharmacological intervention (drugs which increase gastric motility):
  - Domperidone or metoclopramide (act on the dopaminergic receptors):
    - Metoclopramide may cause extrapyramidal side effects with prolonged use.
    - Recent EU review has produced new recommendations on use of metoclopramide (see MICRO-facts box below).
    - With domperidone, 5% of patients develop symptomatic hyperprolactinaemia.

- Recently, the EU has advised that use of domperidone is contraindicated in patients with certain cardiac conditions.
  - Erythromycin (stimulates motilin receptors).
- Botox: injected into pylorus at endoscopy results in temporary paralysis of the pylorus keeping it open for longer to aid emptying.
- Surgical:
  - Gastric pacemaker (paces distal stomach at a high-frequency 12 contractions per minute).
  - Jejunostomy (endoscopic or surgical).
  - Gastric bypass/resection.

COMPLICATIONS

- Bacterial overgrowth in stomach.
- Bezoar (solid mass of undigested food in stomach).
- Unstable blood sugars levels secondary to problems absorbing food.
- Malnutrition.

MICRO-facts

The European Medicines Agency (EMA) has issued new recommendations for prescribing metoclopramide due to the neurological side effects associated with its use.

Recommendations include restricting prescription of metoclopramide to a maximum of 5 days.

For more information, see: http://www.ema.europa.eu/ema/index.jsp?curl=pages/news_and_events/news/2013/07/news_detail_001854.jsp&mid=WC0b01ac058004d5c1

6.7 GASTRIC CANCER

EPIDEMIOLOGY

- The fourth most common cancer worldwide and the second most common cause of cancer death after lung cancer.
- The 13th most common cancer in the UK and the seventh most common cause of cancer death.
- UK incidence is around 8 per 100,000.
- Worldwide incidence is falling.
- More common in males than females (1.8:1).
- Risk increases with age.
- Histopathological grouping:
  - Adenocarcinoma accounts for 90% of gastric cancers.
  - Lymphomas account for approximately a further 5%.

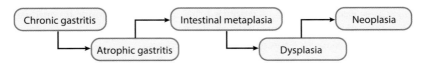

Figure 6.2 Pathophysiology of gastric cancer.

- Rare tumours make up the remaining 5%:
  - Carcinoid tumours.
  - GIST (gastrointestinal stromal tumours).

RISK FACTORS

- *H. pylori* infection.
- Dietary factors:
  - High salt and nitrate intake increases risk by the conversion of nitrates to carcinogenic nitrosamines.
  - Fruit and vegetables are protective: antioxidants.
- Smoking.
- Blood group A.
- Achlorhydria/hypochlorhydria: reduces acid levels allowing proliferation of bacteria.
- Post-partial gastrectomy.
- Pernicious anaemia.
- Ménétrier's disease.
- Family history.

PATHOPHYSIOLOGY

- *H. pylori* is a common cause of chronic corpus gastritis:
  - Prevalence of *H. pylori* is related to incidence of gastric cancer:
    - 1/3 of gastric cancers in the UK are related to *H. pylori*.
    - Associated with both adenocarcinoma and lymphoma.
- *H. pylori* oncogenic mechanisms:
  - Chronic inflammation of the gastric corpus leads to glandular atrophy resulting in reduced acid secretion. Elevated gastric pH allows growth of nitrate-reducing bacteria, producing nitrites which are subsequently converted to carcinogenic *N*-nitroso compounds.
  - Chronic inflammation by *H. pylori* attracts neutrophils which produce free radicals such as superoxide and hydroxyl ions resulting in DNA damage.
  - Increased cell turnover compromises DNA repair.
- The majority of lesions occur in the proximal stomach.

- Tumour types:
  - Polypoidal.
  - Ulcerated.
  - Diffuse: linitis plastica:
    - Leather bottle stomach: hard, thickened and small.
- Tumour suppressor genes lost: p53 (70%), APC (50%), k-Ras (15%).

MICRO-facts

Benign and malignant stomach ulcers are difficult to differentiate during endoscopy. All stomach ulcers should be biopsied to rule out malignancy.

CLINICAL FEATURES

- History:
  - Early satiety.
  - Nausea/vomiting: loss of gastric compliance/gastric outflow obstruction.
  - Weight loss.
  - Abdominal pain/dyspepsia.
  - Melaena.
  - Metastatic symptoms: ascites, jaundice.
- Examination:
  - Epigastric pain/dyspepsia.
  - Cachexia.
  - Epigastric mass: suggestive of advanced disease.
  - Virchow's node: enlarged lymph node in left supraclavicular fossa.
  - Sister Joseph's nodule: metastasis in umbilicus producing a palpable node.
  - Paraneoplastic syndromes:
    - Dermatomyositis: connective tissue disease with muscle and skin inflammation.
    - Acanthosis nigricans: velvety hyperpigmentation of the skin, usually in the folds.

INVESTIGATIONS

- OGD: biopsy of lesion and therapeutic intervention.
- Barium meal (rarely carried out).
- Blood tests: FBC, LFTs.
- CT scan/PET/endoscopic ultrasound/laparoscopy used to stage the tumour.
- TNM staging (see MICRO-reference box in Section 5.7).

MANAGEMENT

- Endoscopic treatment:
  - For early cancers confined to the mucosa.

Gastroenterology

- Two techniques available for removal of the affected mucosa:
  - Endoscopic mucosal resection (EMR).
  - Endoscopic submucosal dissection (ESD).
- Surgery:
  - Curative:
    - For tumours which have invaded the submucosa but have not spread beyond the stomach.
    - Total/subtotal gastrectomy.
  - Palliative:
    - Endoscopic stenting of the pylorus to maintain gastric outflow tract or stenting of the gastro-oesophageal junction for proximal lesions.
    - Surgical bypass.
- Chemotherapy and radiotherapy:
  - Adjuvant chemotherapy considered for patients with a high risk of recurrence.
  - Palliative chemotherapy using multiple agents (epirubicin, cisplatin, 5-FU) may prolong survival.

COMPLICATIONS

- Obstruction of gastric outflow.
- Upper GI haemorrhage.

PROGNOSIS

- Overall 5-year survival rate: around 17–18%.
- Early diagnosed cancers (T1) have a 5-year survival rate of around 90%.
- Most cancers are advanced when diagnosis is made:
  - Curative surgery only possible in 1/3.

MICRO-case

A 59-year-old woman is brought to the ED following a collapse. The paramedics report signs that the patient has been vomiting blood. Upon initial examination, the junior doctor finds the patient to be pale with subconjunctival pallor. She is tachycardic with a pulse of 120 bpm and a systolic blood pressure of 82 mmHg. Her abdomen is soft and non-tender. A quick review of the patient's previous hospital notes shows that the patient had previously undergone endoscopic therapy for a bleeding peptic ulcer 3 years earlier. The junior doctor inserts two large bore cannulas into the ante-cubital fossae and takes blood tests, including FBC, clotting, U&Es and cross-matches 4 units of blood. The doctor starts the patient on a crystalloid infusion awaiting type-specific blood and informs his or her senior of the patient's condition. The patient's FBC returns: haemoglobin 72 g/L, WCC 8.0×10^9/L, Plts 455×10^9/L.

continued...

Gastroenterology

continued...

The patient starts to become increasingly delirious, sweaty and more tachycardic. The junior doctor realizes the patient is developing hypovolaemic shock and orders 4 units of O Rh –ve blood and makes an urgent referral to the on-call endoscopist. The patient is transfused 2 units of blood and regains consciousness and her systolic blood pressure increases to 100 mmHg. She is taken to the endoscopy unit where she is found to have a bleeding gastric ulcer. This is treated by injection of adrenaline and heater probe, and the patient is started on intravenous PPI and transferred to the high dependency unit.

Once the patient is stable, the junior doctor takes a full medical history and learns that the patient has recently begun a prescription of naproxen from her GP to alleviate the severe pain caused by her migraines.

Key points:

- In severe cases, actively bleeding peptic ulcers may present with signs of shock.
- Such cases require urgent referral for endoscopic haemostasis following resuscitation.
- Large volume transfusions require simultaneous transfusion of platelets and clotting factors.
- Scoring systems such as the Blatchford Score allows assessment of the severity of cases and should be performed for all cases (see Section 1.3).
- The use of non-selective NSAIDs are contraindicated in patients with a history of peptic ulcer disease.
- NICE recommend starting IV PPI in patients with high-risk ulcers following endoscopy.

The small bowel

7.1 ANATOMY

MUSCLE LAYERS

- Similar to the rest of the GI tract, the wall of the small bowel is composed of two muscle layers (circular and longitudinal):
  - These run just under the outer surface, beneath the serosa (see Figure 7.1).
  - The myenteric plexus is located between the two muscle layers.
- Inside the muscular layers is the submucosa:
  - This consists of the submucosal nerve plexus as well as blood and lymphatic vessels in a layer of connective tissue.
- The innermost layer is called the mucosa and consists of several parts:
  - The muscularis mucosa – a thin layer of muscle.
  - The lamina propria – a layer of connective tissue with small blood and lymphatic vessels along with nerve fibres.
  - The epithelium – the lining of the small bowel containing cells specialized for their absorptive, transport, secretory and barrier functions.

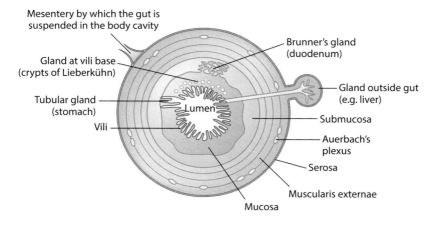

Figure 7.1 Anatomy of the small bowel.

MECHANISMS OF INCREASING ABSORPTION

- Maximizing surface area – the small bowel is adapted in several ways which increase surface area by around 600 times compared to a flat mucosa:
  - Folds – the mucosa is folded.
  - Villi – finger-like projections of the mucosa into the lumen.
  - Microvilli (brush border) – finger-like projections of the apical portion of the enterocytes into the lumen (increase surface area by 20 times).
- Good blood supply:
  - A network of blood vessels runs inside the villi rapidly removing absorbed nutrients.
- Good lymphatic drainage:
  - A blind-ended lymphatic vessel called a lacteal runs inside each villus.
  - Removes absorbed fat in the form of chylomicrons (fat and protein compounds) from the villi.

7.2 PHYSIOLOGY

FUNCTIONS

- Digestion:
  - Mechanical: muscle contractions mix and divide contents.
  - Enzymatic:
    - Brush border enzymes:
      - o Oligosaccharidases/disaccharidases: break down larger sugars into monosaccharidases.
      - o Aminopeptidases: break down small peptides.
    - Pancreatic enzymes:
      - o Amylase: breaks down starch.
      - o Lipases: break down fats.
      - o Proteases: break down proteins.
  - Other:
    - Bile: emulsifies fats to increase the area for enzymatic digestion.
- Absorption:
  - Fluid balance:
    - 9 litres of fluid enter small bowel daily.
    - 7 litres are absorbed by the small bowel.
  - Nutrient absorption:
    - Enterocytes specialized for absorption of digested nutrients:
      - o Transporter proteins allow facilitated diffusion or active transport.
    - Good blood supply and lymphatic drainage to remove absorbed nutrients.

- Defence:
  - Areas of lymphoid tissue are present in walls of small bowel:
    - Mucosa-associated lymphoid tissue (MALT).
    - Mainly composed of CD4 and CD8 lymphocytes.

CONTROL OF DIGESTION

- See Table 7.1 for small bowel physiology.

Table 7.1 **Small bowel physiology**

SECRETION	CELL OF PRODUCTION	STIMULUS	ROLE
Gastrin	Antral G cells	Amino acids or peptides in stomach	Stimulates stomach motility and acid secretion. Stimulates ileal and colonic motility.
Cholecystikinin (CCK)	Duodenal endocrine cells	Amino acids and fatty acids in small intestine	Inhibits stomach motility and acid secretion. Stimulates pancreatic enzyme secretion. Potentiates secretin's actions. Stimulates gallbladder contraction and relaxes the sphincter of Oddi.
Secretin	Duodenal S cells	Acid in small intestine	Inhibits stomach motility and acid secretion. Stimulates bicarbonate production from the pancreas and bile ducts of the liver. Potentiates CCK's actions.
Glucose-dependent insulinotropic peptide (GIP)	K cells of small intestinal mucosa	Glucose and fat in small intestine	Stimulates insulin secretion from the pancreas.
Somatostatin	Antral, small intestinal and pancreatic D cells	Glucose, amino acids and fatty acids in small intestine	Inhibits insulin, glucagon, pepsin, secretin and gastrin secretion. Decreases motility of stomach, gall bladder and duodenum.

Gastroenterology

7.3 COELIAC DISEASE

DEFINITION

- A T-cell immune response to ingestion of gluten-containing cereal grains in a genetically predisposed individual resulting in chronic inflammation of the small intestine leading to mucosal atrophy and malabsorption.

EPIDEMIOLOGY

- Prevalence of 1 in 100 in UK.
- Lower prevalence in Asia and Africa.
- Female to male ratio is 3:1.
- Two peaks of incidence: early childhood and around the fifth decade.

AETIOLOGY

- Coeliac disease occurs in genetically susceptible individuals:
  - 10–15% of sufferers will have an affected first-degree relative.
  - Associated with two human leukocyte antigen (HLA) groups:
    - HLA DQ2 – 90% of sufferers will have this HLA type.
    - HLA DQ8.
    - If patients do not have either of these HLA types, then coeliac disease is extremely unlikely.
  - Other genetic changes have been implicated but are less well understood.
- Associated with:
  - Dermatitis herpetiformis – 90% have villous atrophy.
  - Microscopic colitis.
  - Type 1 diabetes mellitus – 3–8% have coeliac disease.
  - Other autoimmune diseases (Addison's disease, thyroid disease, Sjögren's syndrome, SLE, polymyositis, primary biliary cirrhosis).
  - Down's syndrome and Turner's syndrome.

PATHOPHYSIOLOGY

- Gluten is a protein found in wheat, rye and barley:
  - Gluten-containing peptides include gliadins from wheat, secalins from rye and hordeins from barley.
  - All are toxic in coeliac disease, but some are more damaging than others.

- Affected individuals mount an inflammatory response to gliadins in the small intestinal mucosa (see Figure 7.2):
  - T-cell mediated.
  - Inflammation causes changes in the structure of the mucosa:
    - Villous atrophy.
    - Crypt hyperplasia.
    - Chronic inflammatory cells in mucosa.
    - Increased intra-epithelial lymphocytes.
  - Proximal small intestine is worst affected region.
- Malabsorption occurs:
  - Secondary to the reduction in surface area.
  - See Section 2.1 for details on malabsorption.

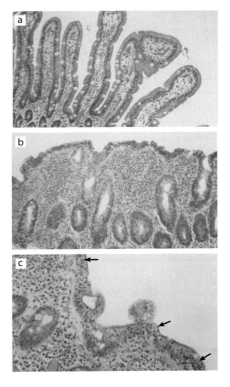

Figure 7.2 Duodenal biopsies showing coeliac disease. (a) Normal duodenal biopsy. (b) Villous atrophy and crypt hyperplasia on a duodenal biopsy from a patient with coeliac disease. (c) Increased intra-epithelial lymphocytes (arrows) in the duodenal mucosa.

CLINICAL FEATURES

- History:
    - Diarrhoea: only occurs in 50% and some patients may be constipated.
    - Steatorrhoea.
    - Abdominal discomfort/bloating/pain.
- Extra-intestinal manifestations:
    - Failure to thrive in children.
    - Tiredness.
    - Malaise.
    - Weight loss.
- Examination:
    - In children:
        - Buttock wasting.
        - Abdominal distension.
    - General:
        - Anaemia: iron deficiency.
        - Mouth ulcers.
        - Angular stomatitis.
        - Osteoporosis/fractures.
    - Dermatitis herpetiformis:
        - Itchy, vesicular rash commonly occurring on elbows, knees, scalp and buttocks.
    - Rarely neurological symptoms may occur as a result of systemic involvement/nutrient deficiency:
        - Cerebellar ataxia.
        - Paraesthesia secondary to peripheral neuropathy.
        - Muscle weakness.

MICRO-print

There may be a role for wireless capsule endoscopy in assessing patients for complications of coeliac disease or in patients suffering from persistent or recurrent symptoms on a gluten-free diet.

INVESTIGATIONS

- Blood tests:
    - FBC, vitamin B_{12}, folate, ferritin, calcium, phosphate, vitamin D, PTH, LFTs, TFTs.

- Immunology:
  - Tissue transglutaminase antibodies (tTG) and endomysial antibodies (EMA):
    - IgA antibodies.
    - tTG is first line while EMA is used if tTG is unavailable or gives an equivocal result.
    - tTG is sensitive (98%) but not specific (90–94%) for coeliac disease.
    - EMA is less sensitive (around 90%) but more specific (98%).
    - Patients need to remain on a gluten-containing diet when samples are taken.
    - Levels of tTG and EMA fall on a gluten-free diet and usual become negative. Useful for monitoring compliance.
  - IgA deficiency:
    - 0.4% of the population and 2.6% of patients with coeliac disease are IgA deficient.
    - Can provide false-negative results.
    - IgG EMA and tTG antibodies should be tested in these patients.
  - HLA typing:
    - Should be reserved for patients with an equivocal diagnosis.
- Endoscopy:
  - Although often macroscopically normal, certain changes in the macroscopic appearance of the mucosa may be seen:
    - Scalloping, mosaic pattern, nodular pattern, prominent submucosal blood vessels, paucity of folds.
  - Biopsy:
    - Several biopsies taken from duodenum or jejunum.
    - Histology of these biopsies uses the Marsh grading system.
- DEXA bone scan: to exclude osteoporosis.

MICRO-references
Sidu R, Sanders DS, Morris AJ, et al. Guidelines on small bowel enteroscopy and capsule endoscopy in adults. *Gut* 2008; 57: 125–136.
   For further information on the Marsh grading system for coeliac disease, see: http://surgpathcriteria.stanford.edu/gi/celiac-disease/marsh.html

---

MANAGEMENT

- Lifelong gluten-free diet.
- Treatment of anaemia: iron, folic acid.
- Pneumococcal vaccination due to splenic atrophy (see Section 7.3).

Gastroenterology

MICRO-facts

Foods acceptable as part of a gluten-free diet:
- Potatoes
- Rice
- Oats
- Soya
- Maize

Foods to avoid:
- Wheat
- Barley
- Rye

MICRO-facts

Alcoholic drinks acceptable as part of a gluten-free diet:
- Wine
- Gin
- Rum
- Whiskey
- Brandy
- Cider

Alcoholic drinks to avoid:
- Most beer (gluten-free varieties are available)

COMPLICATIONS

- Malabsorption and associated complications (see Section 2.1).
- Lymphoma:
  - Enteropathy associated T-cell lymphoma is more common in patients with coeliac disease than in the general public.
  - Other non-Hodgkin's lymphomas are also more common.
- Carcinoma:
  - Increased incidence of small bowel and oesophageal carcinomas.
  - Other extra-intestinal cancers may be more common (e.g. pancreas).
- Splenic atrophy.
- Refractory symptoms:
  - Failure to respond is usually secondary to ongoing gluten exposure.
  - Other possible causes include concomitant problems such as:
    - Microscopic colitis.
    - Pancreatic insufficiency.
    - Hypolactasia.

- Refractory sprue:
  - Patients with persisting symptoms in the presence of villous atrophy despite adherence to a gluten-free diet for 6–12 months are said to have refractory sprue.
  - Patients with type 2 refractory disease, characterized by clonal expansion of intra-epithelial lymphocytes, are at increased risk of complications such as lymphoma or ulcerative jejunitis.

7.4 WHIPPLE'S DISEASE

DEFINITION

- A rare bacterial infection, usually of the small bowel, caused by *Tropheryma whipplei* leading to intestinal and systemic symptoms.

RISK FACTORS

- Much more common in white, middle-aged males.
- Familial clustering: patients may be genetically susceptible.
- More common in patients who work with sewage or in farmers.

CLINICAL FEATURES

- History:
  - Diarrhoea.
  - Steatorrhoea.
  - Abdominal pain.
  - Abdominal distension.
- Extra-intestinal symptoms:
  - Fever.
  - Weight loss.
  - Arthralgia:
    - Chronic, affects mainly peripheral joints.
  - Skin hyperpigmentation.
  - CNS involvement: headache, confusion, dementia.
  - Chronic cough.
  - Cardiac involvement:
    - Chest pain secondary to pericarditis or myocarditis.
- Examination:
  - Lymphadenopathy.
  - Anaemia.
  - CNS involvement: ophthalmoplegia, myoclonus, gait abnormalities.
  - Ocular involvement: uveitis, retinitis, retinal haemorrhages.
  - Pulmonary involvement: pleural effusion.
  - Cardiac involvement: pericarditis, endocarditis.

Gastroenterology

INVESTIGATIONS

- Endoscopy:
    - Small bowel biopsy:
        - Periodic acid–Schiff (PAS) stain shows PAS-positive macrophages with intracellular *T. whippelii* in lamina propria.
        - Stunted villi.
- Polymerase chain reaction (PCR) for *T. whippelii*:
    - Peripheral blood, CSF or other affected tissue sample.

MANAGEMENT

- Antibiotic therapy:
    - Must be able to cross blood–brain barrier (consult with microbiology).
    - Induction therapy: IV antibiotics for 2 weeks (e.g. ceftriaxone).
    - Maintenance therapy: oral antibiotics for 1 year (e.g. co-trimoxazole).

PROGNOSIS

- Usually rapid improvement with treatment.
- Relapse:
    - May be refractory to repeat treatment.
    - Therefore can cause severe neurological complications and even death.

7.5 SMALL INTESTINE BACTERIAL OVERGROWTH

DEFINITION

- Overgrowth of bacteria in small bowel resulting in malabsorption.

AETIOLOGY

- Usually secondary to structural abnormality of the small bowel:
    - Obstruction: secondary to strictures resulting from IBD or surgery.
    - Post-surgical diversion: also called blind loop syndrome.
    - Jejunal diverticulosis.
    - Fistulae: can occur in patients with Crohn's disease.
    - Resection/dysfunction of the ileocaecal valve allowing retrograde migration of colonic bacteria.
- Can be secondary to stasis in a structurally normal small bowel:
    - Diabetes mellitus (and other autonomic dysfunction).
    - Scleroderma.
    - Post radiotherapy.
- Immunosuppression: inherited conditions, immunosuppressive medications.
- Can occasionally be found in otherwise healthy elderly patients.

> **MICRO-print**
> There is a possible link between SIBO and irritable bowel syndrome (IBS). A meta-analysis in 2004 estimated that almost 80% of IBS patients may have SIBO and therefore may benefit from treatment.
>   Lin HC. Small intestinal bacterial overgrowth: a framework for understanding irritable bowel syndrome. *JAMA* 2004; 292(7): 852–858.

PATHOPHYSIOLOGY

- The bacteria colonizing the small bowel in SIBO are normal gut flora:
    - Usually found only in the colon and terminal ileum.
    - Common species include: *Escherichia coli, Bacteroides, Enterococci, Lactobacilli, Streptococci.*

CLINICAL FEATURES

- History:
    - Diarrhoea.
    - Steatorrhoea – secondary to bacterial metabolism of bile salts, leading to malabsorption of fat-soluble vitamins.
    - Abdominal bloating.
- Vitamin B_{12} deficiency – secondary to bacterial metabolism of vitamin B_{12} which interferes with its binding to intrinsic factor.

INVESTIGATIONS

- Hydrogen breath test:
    - Hydrogen is produced when orally ingested lactulose or glucose is metabolized by bacteria.
    - Early production of hydrogen suggests SIBO but may also indicate fast transit of lactulose/glucose into the large bowel.
- Radioisotope breath tests:
    - Uses a radioactive isotope of carbon incorporated into a larger molecule.
    - ^{14}C released and detected in breath sample.
    - Rarely used – largely replaced by hydrogen breath test.
- Small bowel aspirate:
    - Gold standard test although not routinely carried out.
    - More than 10^5 bacteria per millilitre is diagnostic.

MANAGEMENT

- Treatment of any underlying structural pathology if possible.
- Antibiotics:
    - Metronidazole/tetracycline/ciprofloxacin are commonly used for 2 weeks and then repeated if symptoms return.

Gastroenterology

7.6 GASTROINTESTINAL INFECTIONS

Table 7.2 **Microbiology table**

PATHOGEN	INCUBATION	MECHANISM	DURATION	TRANSMISSION	SYMPTOMS AND DIAGNOSIS	TREATMENT
Bacteria						
Staphylococcus aureus	2–4 hours (toxin preformed → rapid onset)	Enterotoxin B → intestinal fluid secretion	24 hours	• Food borne • Poor food hygiene, e.g. food handler with infected hand lesion	• Initially vomiting and abdominal pain; later diarrhoea • Dehydration • **Diagnosis:** culture from vomit or food	• Fluid replacement • Supportive
Shigella spp.	1–2 days	Mucosal cell invasion and destruction → diarrhoea with blood and abdominal pain	5–7 days	• Faecal–oral • Small number of organisms can cause illness	• Dysentery (diarrhoea with blood and mucus) • Fever and abdominal pain • **Complications:** toxic megacolon (rare) and HUS • **Diagnosis:** stool culture	• Fluid replacement • Supportive • Ciprofloxacin or amoxicillin or trimethoprim

(Continued)

Table 7.2 (Continued) **Microbiology table**

PATHOGEN	INCUBATION	MECHANISM	DURATION	TRANSMISSION	SYMPTOMS AND DIAGNOSIS	TREATMENT
Salmonella spp.	8–48 hours	Enterotoxin → intestinal fluid secretion	4–7 days	• Faecal–oral • Commensals of poultry • Contamination of red and white meat, raw eggs and dairy products	• Bloody watery diarrhoea • Nausea and vomiting • Fever • Abdominal pain • Headache • **Diagnosis:** stool or blood culture (rarely used)	• Fluid replacement • Supportive • Ciprofloxacin (decreases severity and duration but rarely used)
Campylobacter spp.	2–5 days	Mucosal cell invasion and toxin production	5–7 days	• Faecal–oral • Commensal of livestock • Contamination of undercooked meat (poultry), water and milk	• Diarrhoea (profuse and occasionally bloody) • Nausea and vomiting • Abdominal pain • Fever • **Complications:** Guillain–Barré syndrome • **Diagnosis:** stool culture	• Fluid replacement • Supportive • Erythromycin or azithromycin (severe cases)

(*Continued*)

Gastroenterology

Table 7.2 (Continued) **Microbiology table**

PATHOGEN	INCUBATION	MECHANISM	DURATION	TRANSMISSION	SYMPTOMS AND DIAGNOSIS	TREATMENT
Escherichia coli • Enteroinvasive *E. coli* (EIEC)	• Shigellosis-like disease • **Diagnosis**: stool culture					
• Enterotoxigenic *E. coli* (ETEC)	1–2 days	Enterotoxin → intestinal fluid secretion	2–3 days	• Faecal–oral • Contamination of water and food • Common cause of traveller's diarrhoea	• Diarrhoea (watery)	• Fluid replacement • Supportive
• Enterohaemorrhagic (EHEC)/verotoxin-producing *E. coli* (VTEC)	12–48 hours	Serotype O157:H7 secretes Shiga-like toxin 1 → damage of gut and renal endothelial cells	2–3 days	• Faecal–oral • Contamination of water and food • Commensal of cattle	• Diarrhoea (commonly bloody). • Abdominal pain • Nausea • **Complications**: HUS (7–10 days later) • **Diagnosis**: stool culture	• Fluid replacement • Supportive • HUS: admit to hospital • Avoid antibiotics as may precipitate HUS

(Continued)

Table 7.2 (*Continued*) **Microbiology table**

PATHOGEN	INCUBATION	MECHANISM	DURATION	TRANSMISSION	SYMPTOMS AND DIAGNOSIS	TREATMENT
Vibrio cholerae	1–6 days	Enterotoxin → intestinal fluid secretion	<1 week	• Faecal–oral • Contamination of water and food • Associated with poor hygiene standards, e.g. refugee camps	• Spectrum of diarrhoeal illness • Mild diarrhoea to profuse watery diarrhoea (>25 litres 'rice water' stool per day) • Severe dehydration • **Diagnosis:** clinical, stool culture or microscopy	• Oral/intravenous fluid replacement • Tetracycline reduces time of excretion, therefore reducing risk of transmission
Clostridium perfringens	8–24 hours	Enterotoxin → intestinal fluid secretion	1 day	• Spores replicate in red/white meat allowed to cool	• Diarrhoea (watery) • Nausea and vomiting • Abdominal pain	• Fluid replacement • Supportive

(*Continued*)

Table 7.2 (Continued) **Microbiology table**

PATHOGEN	INCUBATION	MECHANISM	DURATION	TRANSMISSION	SYMPTOMS AND DIAGNOSIS	TREATMENT
Clostridium difficile	Days to months after antibiotics	Enterotoxin (toxin A) → intestinal fluid secretion and cytotoxin (toxin B) → cell damage	Variable	• Normal bowel commensal in 3–5% population • Antibiotics eliminate other bowel flora → *C. difficile* infection • Faecal–oral transmission can occur • Common antibiotics include clindamycin and cephalosporins • Linked to poor hand hygiene in hospitals	• Spectrum of diarrhoeal illness • Mild diarrhoeal illness to pseudomembranous colitis (haemorrhagic colitis, diarrhoea and abdominal pain with colonic pseudomembrane) • Can be fatal in elderly patients • **Diagnosis**: ELISA detection of toxins in stools	• Fluid replacement • Discontinue causative antibiotics • Metronidazole or vancomycin

(Continued)

Table 7.2 (Continued) **Microbiology table**

PATHOGEN	INCUBATION	MECHANISM	DURATION	TRANSMISSION	SYMPTOMS AND DIAGNOSIS	TREATMENT
Clostridium botulinum	1–2 days	Neurotoxin → paralysis	2–3 weeks	• Spores contaminate preserved/ tinned foods, replicate and produce neurotoxin • Neurotoxin ingested with food	• Diarrhoea • Paralysis • Respiratory muscle paralysis can be fatal • **Diagnosis:** detect toxin in stool sample or food	• Supportive • Antitoxin
Bacillus cereus	**Vomiting form:** 2–5 hours (toxin preformed) **Diarrhoea form:** 10–12 hours	Produces two toxins → vomiting or diarrhoea	12–24 hours	• **Vomiting:** spores survive, multiply and produce a toxin in rice left to cool for a long time • **Diarrhoea:** ice cream or meat	• Vomiting • Diarrhoea • Abdominal pain • **Diagnosis:** stool culture	• Fluid replacement • Supportive

(Continued)

Table 7.2 (*Continued*) **Microbiology table**

PATHOGEN	INCUBATION	MECHANISM	DURATION	TRANSMISSION	SYMPTOMS AND DIAGNOSIS	TREATMENT
Viruses						
Rotavirus	2–3 days	Cell destruction and intestinal fluid secretion	3–9 days	• Faecal–oral • Environmental contamination • Common in children; adults develop lifelong resistance	• Fever • Vomiting • Diarrhoea • **Diagnosis**: virus isolation in cell culture from stool sample	• Fluid replacement • Supportive
Norovirus	1–2 days	Cell destruction	1–2 days	• Faecal–oral • Contaminates food, water or environmental surfaces	• Nausea and vomiting • Diarrhoea (watery) • Fever • Headache • Aching limbs	• Fluid replacement • Supportive
Adenovirus	3–10 days	Infection of intestinal epithelial cells	1–2 days	• Faecal–oral	• Diarrhoea • **Diagnosis**: virus isolation in cell culture from stool sample	• Fluid replacement • Supportive

(*Continued*)

Table 7.2 (Continued) **Microbiology table**

PATHOGEN	INCUBATION	MECHANISM	DURATION	TRANSMISSION	SYMPTOMS AND DIAGNOSIS	TREATMENT
Protozoa						
Giardia lamblia	7–21 days	Trophozoites attach to intestinal villi → inflammation	Variable	• Faecal–oral • Cysts contaminate water or food	• Asymptomatic carrier • Diarrhoea (slimy and foul smelling) • Abdominal pain • Nausea and vomiting • Malabsorption • Bloating and excessive flatus • **Diagnosis:** microscopy of stool sample	• Fluid replacement • Supportive • Metronidazole
Cryptosporidium parvum	3–6 days	Sporozoites invade intestinal epithelium → inflammation	Several weeks; longer in immunocompromised	• Faecal–oral • Infective cysts contaminate water	• Asymptomatic carrier • Diarrhoea (mild) • More severe disease in immunocompromised patients, typically HIV/AIDS • **Diagnosis:** microscopy of stool sample	• Fluid replacement • Supportive

(Continued)

Table 7.2 *(Continued)* **Microbiology table**

PATHOGEN	INCUBATION	MECHANISM	DURATION	TRANSMISSION	SYMPTOMS AND DIAGNOSIS	TREATMENT
Entamoeba histolytica	Variable, days to months	Multiplication of trophozoites in the colon can cause inflammation and necrosis	Chronic unless treated	• Faecal–oral. • Infective cysts contaminate water or food	• Chronic mild diarrhoea • Abdominal pain • Later, bloody diarrhoea • Nausea • Headache • **Complications**: toxic megacolon, strictures and liver abscesses • **Diagnosis**: microscopy of stool sample	• Fluid replacement • Supportive • Metronidazole or tinidazole

AIDS, acquired immune deficiency syndrome; ELISA, enzyme-linked immunosorbent assay; HIV, human immunodeficiency virus; HUS, haemolytic uraemic syndrome.

7.7 LACTOSE INTOLERANCE

DEFINITION

- Deficiency of the brush border enzyme lactase, leading to decreased digestion of lactose, a disaccharide found in milk and dairy products.
- Classification:
  - Acquired primary – common genetic condition.
  - Secondary – caused by damage to small bowel mucosa, commonly following gastroenteritis; resolves once causative factor is removed.
  - Congenital – rare autosomal recessive disorder.
  - Developmental – occurs in babies born at <34 weeks' gestation and improves as intestine fully develops.

EPIDEMIOLOGY

- The prevalence of primary lactose intolerance varies according to geographical location:
  - 2% in Northern Europe.
  - Over 90% in some parts of Asia and Africa.
  - Overall worldwide prevalence is between 70% and 80%.

PATHOPHYSIOLOGY

- Lactase is an enzyme on the brush border of the small intestinal villi:
  - Hydrolyzes lactose (disaccharide) into glucose and galactose (monosaccharides).
- The lack of lactase means lactose can pass through the small bowel undigested:
  - Metabolized by colonic bacteria in a process that produces large amounts of gas (methane, carbon dioxide and hydrogen).
  - Unabsorbed sugars alter the osmotic gradient across the colon leading to an influx of water into the bowels.
- Acquired primary lactose intolerance:
  - Most begin life with normal lactase activity that decreases at the time of weaning and continues to decrease throughout childhood/adulthood.
  - Primary lactose intolerance occurs in those where lactase activity decreases with time due to the absence of the lactose persistence allele.
- Secondary lactose intolerance:
  - Damage to the mucosa reduces the amount of functioning lactase.
  - Gastroenteritis, coeliac disease and chemotherapy can all be causative.
- Congenital lactose intolerance:
  - Autosomal recessive disorder resulting in lack of lactase expression.

Gastroenterology

CLINICAL FEATURES

- History (symptoms tend to appear 1–2 hours after ingestion of lactose):
  - Diarrhoea.
  - Abdominal bloating.
  - Flatulence.
  - Nausea.
  - Borborygmi (rumbling of the stomach).
  - Perianal itching secondary to acidic stools.
- Examination:
  - Malnutrition and failure to thrive in children.

INVESTIGATIONS

- Lactose tolerance test:
  - Dose of lactose (50 g) given after a period of fasting and rise in blood glucose is measured.
  - A rise of less than 1.11 mmol/L is diagnostic.
  - Not commonly used – superseded by breath hydrogen test.
- Breath hydrogen test:
  - Increased hydrogen production by fermentation of lactose by colonic bacteria causes a rise in hydrogen levels, which is exhaled from the lungs.
  - A dose of lactose is given and the breath hydrogen levels are recorded.
- Small bowel biopsy:
  - Not routinely carried out.
  - Biopsy specimen can be tested for lactase activity as well as other enzyme activity.

MANAGEMENT

- Removal of lactose (i.e. all cow's milk) from diet:
  - Small amounts of lactose can usually be tolerated.
  - Milk substitutes can be included instead – e.g. soya milk.
- Lactase enzyme preparations are available although expensive.

7.8 SMALL BOWEL TUMOURS

EPIDEMIOLOGY

- Account for 3–6% of GI tumours.
- Histopathological subtypes:
  - Malignant:
    - Adenocarcinomas account for 40% of small bowel malignancies.
    - Neuroendocrine tumours (including carcinoid tumours) make up 30% of small bowel malignancies.

- Lymphomas account for 10% of small bowel malignancies.
- Sarcomas are less common – the most common is a leiomyosarcoma (smooth muscle tumour).
- Benign:
  - Hamartomas occur in Peutz–Jeghers syndrome.
  - Adenomas.
  - Lipomas.
  - Leiomyomas.
  - Neurofibromas.
  - Haemangiomas.

RISK FACTORS

- Peutz–Jeghers syndrome:
  - Autosomal dominant condition causing multiple benign hamartomas and hyperpigmentation of the lips and oral mucosa.
  - Also associated with cancer of the pancreas, breast, uterus, ovary and testes.
- Familial adenomatous polyposis:
  - 60–90% will have duodenal adenomas.
  - 4–12% lifetime risk of adenocarcinoma.
- Coeliac disease: increases the risk of both T-cell lymphomas and adenocarcinoma.
- Crohn's disease: slightly increases the risk of adenocarcinoma.

PATHOPHYSIOLOGY

- Staging of tumours:
  - Small bowel tumours are staged using the TNM (tumour, nodes, metastases) staging system.

CLINICAL FEATURES

- History:
  - Abdominal pain due to obstruction/intussusception.
  - Diarrhoea.
  - Anorexia.
  - Weight loss.
  - Tiredness secondary to anaemia.
  - Nausea and vomiting.
  - Overt bleeding/melaena.
  - Carcinoid syndrome in metastatic carcinoid disease.
  - Jaundice with periampullary lesions.
- Examination:
  - Anaemia.
  - Palpable abdominal mass.

INVESTIGATIONS

- Biochemistry:
  - Chromogranin A + B: elevated in neuroendocrine tumours.
  - 5-Hydroxyindole acetic acid: elevated in metastatic carcinoid.
  - CEA usually only elevated in metastatic adenocarcinoma.
- Imaging:
  - Small bowel follow-through/enteroclysis (barium delivered down nasojejunal tube to beyond ligament of Treitz).
  - CT scan of the abdomen.
  - Nuclear medicine: octreotide scan for carcinoid tumours.
- Endoscopy:
  - Capsule endoscopy.
  - Double balloon enteroscopy – for biopsy/therapeutic intervention.
  - Laparoscopy/intraoperative endoscopy.

MANAGEMENT

- General:
  - Surgery: appropriate for most cancers (especially adenocarcinomas), although most present late. Tumours of the first and second part of duodenum require pancreaticoduodenectomy. Segmental resection is undertaken for other areas.
  - Radiotherapy: mainly for advanced cancers (especially lymphomas).
  - Chemotherapy: mainly reserved for lymphomas.
- Specific treatments:
  - Octreotide (somatostatin analogue): can slow growth of carcinoid tumours.
  - Imatinib (protein tyrosine kinase inhibitor): used for treatment of gastrointestinal stromal tumours (GISTs).
  - Polypectomy:
    - Mainstay of treatment in Peutz–Jeghers syndrome.
    - ERCP/ampullectomy of tumours affecting the ampulla of Vater.

COMPLICATIONS

- Obstruction:
  - Presents with abdominal pain, distension, vomiting and constipation.
  - Immediate management is with decompression via a nasogastric tube.
  - Later management is surgical:
    - Resection of tumour if possible.
    - Bypass/stenting of tumour if inoperable.

- Intussusception:
  - Invagination of one section of small bowel into a more distal part – similar to a telescope collapsing.
  - The invaginated section may become ischaemic as blood supply is cut off.
  - Causes 1% of obstructions and presents in a similar way.
  - May be accompanied by 'red-currant jelly stool' – blood and mucus mixed into the stool as a result of shedding of the ischaemic mucosa.
  - Delayed treatment can result in perforation of ischaemic bowel.
- Carcinoid syndrome:
  - Occurs in 5% of patients with carcinoid tumours.
  - Serotonin and other vasoactive products are released from carcinoid tumours causing:
    - Facial flushing.
    - Diarrhoea.
    - Vomiting.
    - Hepatomegaly.
    - Thickening and stenosis of the pulmonary and tricuspid valves.
    - Dyspnoea, bronchospasm.
- Metastatic spread:
  - As with any malignancy, there is the potential for metastatic spread of the primary tumour.

PROGNOSIS

- Adenocarcinoma – 5-year survival rate after surgery is around 30%.
- Lymphoma:
  - B-cell – 5-year survival rate is 50–60%.
  - T-cell – 5-year survival rate is 25%.
- Carcinoid tumours:
  - Localized disease – 95% 5-year survival rate.
  - Liver metastases – 70% 5-year survival rate.
- Peutz–Jeghers – the risk of developing any cancer increases with age so that by age 70, the majority of people will develop a malignancy.

MICRO-case

A 45-year-old woman presents to you in a GP surgery with a 1-year history of bloating and diarrhoea. She also complains of increasing fatigue and weight loss. On further questioning, she tells you her stools are hard to flush and tend to float in the toilet. She denies seeing any blood in her stool and describes the bloating as a general discomfort in her abdomen with increased flatulence.

continued…

Gastroenterology

continued...

Her past medical history includes type 1 diabetes mellitus that was diagnosed in her early teens.

On examination, she has a vesicular rash over her elbows and knees and her conjunctivae appear pale. Her abdomen is soft with mild generalized tenderness.

A blood test is arranged which shows a microcytic anaemia and her coeliac disease serology (tTG) is positive. The patient is referred to the gastroenterologists for a gastroscopy with duodenal biopsy to confirm coeliac disease. She asks if she should start a gluten-free diet but is advised to continue eating gluten-containing foods until after the endoscopy. The biopsy result shows increased intra-epithelial lymphocytes, crypt hyperplasia and subtotal villous atrophy (Marsh grade 3b). A diagnosis of coeliac disease is made.

Further blood tests are taken to check the patient's vitamin D levels which are in the deficient range and folic acid which is also low. The patient is started on vitamin D and folate as well as iron supplements.

The patient is advised to commence a gluten-free diet and referred to a dietician. Over the following weeks, her symptoms improve.

Key points:

- Coeliac disease has two peaks of incidence:
  - Classical presentation in young children.
  - Second peak in fifth decade of life.
- Coeliac disease is associated with other autoimmune conditions including type 1 diabetes mellitus.
- It can present with an itchy, vesicular rash called dermatitis herpetiformis.
- Coeliac disease can be diagnosed with immunological tests, but duodenal biopsy is the gold standard test.
- With prolonged untreated coeliac disease, it is common for bone structure to deteriorate. Vitamin D levels should be checked, especially in this age group, and replaced as necessary.
- The only treatment for coeliac disease is a gluten-free diet. Complications (e.g. anaemia) should be treated as appropriate.
- Follow-up is important to assess clinical response and monitor normalization of antibodies and electrolyte imbalances.

8 Colorectal disease

8.1 ANATOMY

GENERAL ANATOMY OF THE COLON

- The large bowel extends from the caecum to the anus (see Figure 8.1).
- It can be subdivided into the following parts:
    - Caecum: intraperitoneal blind pouch.
    - Appendix: has its own mesentery (meso-appendix).
    - Ascending colon.
    - Hepatic flexure: located under the right lobe of the liver.
    - Transverse colon: intraperitoneal structure.
    - Splenic flexure: located next to the spleen and the tail of the pancreas.

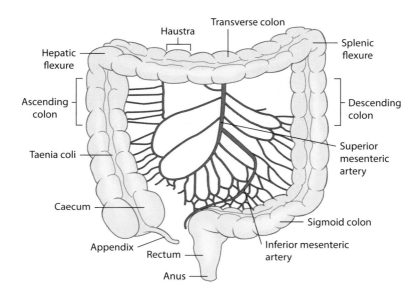

Figure 8.1 Anatomy of the large intestine.

- Descending colon: lies retroperitoneally.
- Sigmoid colon: has a mesentery.
- Rectum.
- Anal canal: extends from the anorectal junction to the anus.

COLONIC STRUCTURE

- The colon consists of four layers:
  - Serosal layer:
    - Derives from the peritoneum and covers different parts of the colon to a variable extent.
  - Muscular layer:
    - Consists of two layers of muscle:
      ○ External longitudinal fibres (produce the haustra).
      ○ Internal circular fibres.
  - Submucosal layer:
    - Connects the muscular layer to the mucosa.
  - Mucosal layer:
    - A smooth, pale coat with no villi.

8.2 IRRITABLE BOWEL SYNDROME

- Affects 5–15% of the population in most developed countries.

DEFINITION

- A relapsing-remitting chronic condition characterized by recurrent abdominal pain, bloating and altered bowel habit.
- Rome III criteria for the diagnosis of irritable bowel syndrome (IBS) require:
  - Recurrent abdominal pain for at least 3 days per month over the past 3 months.
  - Symptoms must have been present for at least 6 months before diagnosis.
  - At least two of the following features:
    - Improvement of pain after defaecation.
    - Change in bowel frequency.

RISK FACTORS

- Female:male ratio of 2:1.
- Family history of IBS.
- Associated psychiatric disorders: depression, anxiety etc.
- Adverse life events.
- Post-infective IBS: 20% have a history of prior gastroenteritis.

PATHOPHYSIOLOGY

- Many mechanisms can lead to IBS:
  - Disturbed bowel motility:
    - Increased high-amplitude propagated contractions in diarrhoea-predominant subtypes.
    - Increase in non-propulsive segmental contractions in constipation-predominant subtypes.
  - Visceral hypersensitivity:
    - Abnormal sensitization within the spinal cord or higher in the CNS.
  - Post-infective IBS (altered gut flora).
  - Stress response.
  - Food intolerance.
  - Local inflammation:
    - Increased number of colonic inflammatory cells including mast cells seen in patients with IBS.

CLINICAL FEATURES

- History:
  - Abdominal pain relieved by defaecation.
  - Frequency of bowel movements (increased or decreased).
  - Bloating.
  - Straining and feeling of incomplete evacuation.
  - Passage of mucus per rectum.
  - Urgency.
  - Altered appearance of stool (form/consistency).
- Examination:
  - May be generalized abdominal tenderness.

MICRO-facts

When taking a history from a patient presenting with features of IBS, red flag symptoms should always be screened for in order to exclude more serious differential diagnoses (indicated in the NICE guidelines below):

- Unintentional weight loss
- Rectal bleeding
- Family history of breast/ovarian cancer
- Change in bowel habit persisting for more than 6 weeks in a patient >60 years of age

continued...

Gastroenterology

continued...

- Abdominal/rectal mass on examination
- Anaemia
- Raised inflammatory markers

NICE clinical guideline 61. Irritable bowel syndrome in adults: Diagnosis and management of irritable bowel syndrome in primary care. February 2008. http://www.nice.org.uk/nicemedia/live/11927/39622/39622.pdf

INVESTIGATIONS

- Blood tests:
  - FBC, coeliac serology (endomysial antibody [EMA] or tissue transglutaminase [tTG]), ESR and CRP.
  - CA-125:
    - Only indicated in women with symptoms suggestive of ovarian cancer.
- Further endoscopic or radiological investigations:
  - Not normally required in patients meeting the Rome III criteria if all other investigations are unremarkable.

MANAGEMENT

- Reassurance.
- Lifestyle advice:
  - Encourage leisure and relaxation time.
  - Encourage physical activity.
- Dietary advice:
  - Regular meals.
  - Minimum of eight glasses of fluid per day.
  - Restriction of alcohol, carbonated drinks and caffeinated drinks.
  - Limit fruit to three portions per day.
  - Avoidance of sorbitol (found in sugar-free drinks and sweets) if patient suffers from predominantly diarrhoea symptoms.
  - Low fermentable oligo-di-monosaccharides and polyol (FODMAP) diet.
- Pharmacological interventions:
  - Symptomatic relief:
    - Laxatives for management of constipation.
    - Loperamide for management of diarrhoea.
    - Anti-spasmodics for pain relief (e.g. mebeverine).
  - Other medications:
    - Tricyclic antidepressants.
- Others:
  - Behavioural management (hypnotherapy, cognitive behavioural therapy).

MICRO-print

The low FODMAP diet has been developed based on poor absorption of the short-chain carbohydrates in the small intestine, which in IBS patients can cause gas production and increase intestinal osmolarity. The FODMAPs in the diet are: fructose (fruits, honey etc.), lactose (dairy), fructans (wheat, garlic, onion, inulin etc.), galactans (legumes such as beans, lentils, soybeans etc.) and polyols (mannitol, sorbitol, xylitol etc.).

A low FODMAP diet may help in reducing global abdominal symptoms presumably due to decrease in the production of hydrogen and methane in the bowel upon minimizing the intake of these short-chain carbohydrates.

Pedersen N, Andersen NN, Véghet Z, et al. Ehealth: low FODMAP diet vs *Lactobacillus rhamnosus* GG in irritable bowel syndrome. *World J Gastroenterol* 2014; 20(43): 16215–16226.

8.3 INFLAMMATORY BOWEL DISEASE

DEFINITION

- Umbrella term for idiopathic chronic conditions of unknown aetiology, characterized by an inflammatory intestinal response to unknown triggers.
- The two major types of inflammatory bowel disease (IBD) are ulcerative colitis (UC) and Crohn's disease (CD) (see Figure 8.2).

EPIDEMIOLOGY

- Incidence of CD is 5–10 cases per 100,000 and UC 10–15 cases per 100,000; increased incidence in Northern latitudes.

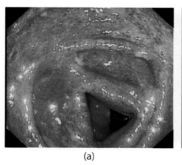 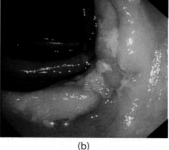

(a)   (b)

Figure 8.2 Colonoscopy images showing (a) ulcerative colitis and (b) Crohn's disease.

Gastroenterology

- Males and females are similarly affected.
- Bimodal age of presentation:
  - Initial peak in the second and third decades of life.
  - Another peak in the sixth decade.

RISK FACTORS

- Family history: greatest independent risk factor.
- Genetic factors: high concordance rate in identical twin studies.
- Poor sanitation/hygiene.
- Smoking: adversely affects the outcome in CD, yet has been shown to reduce hospitalization for UC.
- Poor diet.

CLINICAL FEATURES

- See Sections 8.4 and 8.5 for intestinal features of UC and CD.
- Extra-intestinal features:
  - Dermatological:
    - Erythema nodosum.
    - Pyoderma gangrenosum.
  - Rheumatological:
    - Peripheral (enteropathic) arthropathy.
    - Ankylosing spondylitis (e.g. HLA B27).
  - Ocular:
    - Uveitis.
    - Episcleritis.
  - Metabolic:
    - Osteoporosis.
    - Osteonecrosis.
  - Hepatobiliary:
    - Primary sclerosing cholangitis (PSC).
    - Autoimmune hepatitis.
  - Urological:
    - Calcium oxalate stones.
  - Pulmonary:
    - Interstitial pulmonary fibrosis.
  - Venous and arterial thrombosis.

SCREENING

- Increased risk of bowel cancer in UC and colonic CD.
- Index screening colonoscopy is currently advised for all patients 10 years after the initial diagnosis of IBD.

- Subsequent follow-up is then stratified into 1-, 3- or 5-yearly surveillance according to the presence of associated cancer risks as per the British Society of Gastroenterology (BSG) guideline (e.g. family history of bowel cancer).

8.4 CROHN'S DISEASE

DEFINITION

- Characterized by a discontinuous, trans-mural inflammation that can affect any part of the gastrointestinal (GI) tract.
- Most frequently involves the distal small intestine and proximal colon:
  - Upper GI tract is involved in 0.5–13% of patients.

CLINICAL FEATURES

- History:
  - Diarrhoea.
  - Abdominal pain.
  - Weight loss.
- Examination:
  - Anaemia.
  - Right iliac fossa mass: due to inflamed loops of small bowel or abscess.
  - Fever: due to abscess, acute inflammation or stricture formation.
  - Perianal disease: e.g. abscess, fistula.
  - Mouth ulcers.
  - Associated skin conditions – erythema nodosum, pyoderma gangrenosum.
  - Associated ocular conditions – episcleritis, uveitis, scleritis.

INVESTIGATIONS

- Serological markers:
  - ↑ ESR/CRP.
  - ↑ Platelets.
  - ↓ Albumin (severe disease).
  - ↑ Plasma viscosity.
  - ↑ Plasma orosomucoids.
- Endoscopy:
  - Typical findings are deep ulcers, skip lesions and cobblestone mucosa.

Gastroenterology

- Biopsy:
  - Typical histological findings are non-caseous granulomas, trans-mural involvement and discontinuous inflammation.
- Imaging:
  - Plain abdominal radiograph: small bowel dilatation, mucosal thickening.
  - Small bowel meal: stricture, fistula, erosions, ulcers.
  - MR enterography: bowel wall enhancement, fistula, abscess.
  - CT enteroclysis: mesenteric fibro-fatty proliferation, fistula, abscess, increased bowel wall density, obstruction.
  - Small bowel capsule endoscopy: ≥3 ulcers or >10 aphthous ulcers are suggestive of CD.
- Stool tests:
  - Stool culture: including *Clostridium difficile* toxin.
  - Faecal calprotectin.

MANAGEMENT

- Generally follows a sequential 'step up' approach with more potent drugs or surgery used if initial treatment fails.
- Treatment induction (as per NICE guidance):
  - First presentation:
    - Oral glucocorticoids.
    - Consider enteral nutrition with children/young adults.
    - Consider aminosalicylates in those who cannot tolerate steroids.
    - Consider surgical interventions if medical treatments fail.
  - Severe, active CD:
    - IV corticosteroids.
    - Prophylactic heparin.
    - Add on immunomodulator therapy in patients who do not respond to steroids (infliximab, adalimumab).
    - Consider surgical intervention.
  - Perianal fistulae:
    - Metronidazole/ciprofloxacin.
    - Surgical:
      - Fistulotomy.

MICRO-reference

For full NICE guidance on induction therapy for Crohn's disease, see: http://www.nice.org.uk/guidance/cg152/resources/guidance-crohns-disease-pdf

- Maintenance therapy:
  - Consider maintenance therapy in patients presenting with severe attack or those who have had two or more attacks in a 12-month period:
    - Azathioprine/6-mercaptopurine.
    - Aminosalicylates (alternative to thiopurines for post-surgery maintenance therapy).
    - Methotrexate (if intolerant of thiopurines).
    - Infliximab/adalimumab in those who do not respond to other immunosuppressants or are intolerant of them (assess at 1 year for need to continue).

COMPLICATIONS

- Intestinal complications:
  - Toxic dilatation/perforation.
  - Strictures.
  - Fistulae.
  - Abscess formation.
  - Colorectal carcinoma.
- Opportunistic infections: e.g. *C. difficile* diarrhoea.

8.5 ULCERATIVE COLITIS

DEFINITION

- Chronic inflammatory condition generally affecting the rectum and to a variable extent, the proximal colon in a continuous pattern.
- Only affects the colon, but total colitis may be associated with 'backwash' ileitis.

CLINICAL FEATURES

- History:
  - Bloody diarrhoea.
  - Passage of blood/mucus.
  - Urgency.
  - Abdominal pain.
- Examination:
  - Anaemia.
  - Abdominal tenderness.
  - Fever: due to inflammation ($\uparrow$ pro-inflammatory cytokines).
  - Associated skin conditions – erythema nodosum, pyoderma gangrenosum.
  - Associated ocular conditions – episcleritis, uveitis, scleritis.

Gastroenterology

MICRO-facts

- Truelove–Witts criteria are frequently used in clinical practice for assessing the severity of ulcerative colitis:

ACTIVITY	MILD	MODERATE	SEVERE
No. of stools/day	≤4	4–6	≥6
Rectal bleeding	Small amounts	–	Larger amounts
Fever	No	No	>37.5°C
Tachycardia	No	No	Yes
Anaemia	No	No	Yes (<105 g/L)
ESR	<30 mm/hr	<30 mm/hr	>30 mm/hr

ESR, erythrocyte sedimentation rate.

INVESTIGATIONS

- Serological testing:
  - ↑ ESR/CRP.
  - ↑ Platelets.
  - ↓ Albumin (severe disease).
  - ↑ Plasma viscosity.
  - ↑ Plasma orosomucoids.
- Endoscopy – flexible sigmoidoscopy is the gold standard test:
  - Mucosa appears reddened with loss of the vascular pattern.
  - Either bleeds on contact with the endoscope or has evidence of spontaneous bleeding.
  - Ulcers seen in severe disease.
- Imaging:
  - AXR: mucosal thickening, dilatation, toxic megacolon.
  - Barium enema – mucosal erosion/ulceration, pseudopolyps, cancer:
    - Rarely used for investigation of IBD in modern practice.
  - Abdominal CT:
    - Limited applicability in uncomplicated UC.
    - Useful in excluding differential diagnoses as well as diagnosing suspected UC complications.
- Biopsy:
  - Crypt abscesses.
  - Basal plasmacytosis.
  - Epithelial neutrophil infiltration (inflammation limited to the mucosa).
  - Erosions or ulcerations.

- Stool testing:
  - Stool culture: including *C. difficile* toxin.
  - Faecal calprotectin.

MANAGEMENT

- Treatment induction (as per NICE guidance):
  - Topical therapies usually used initially for distal disease.
    - Mild/moderate colitis:
      - ○ Topical/oral aminosalicylates.
      - ○ Topical/oral corticosteroids.
    - Severe colitis:
      - ○ IV corticosteroids.
      - ○ Prophylactic heparin.
      - ○ IV ciclosporin.
      - ○ Consider surgical options.

> **MICRO-reference**
>
> For full NICE guidelines on induction therapy for ulcerative colitis, see:
> http://www.nice.org.uk/guidance/cg166/resources/guidance-ulcerative-colitis-pdf

- Maintenance therapy:
  - Oral aminosalicylates (first-line maintenance therapy):
    - Intermittent rectal aminosalicylate is effective for maintenance of proctitis and proctosigmoiditis.
  - Azathioprine or mercaptopurine should be considered for maintaining remission in the following circumstances:
    - Patient has had two or more UC flare-ups requiring steroid therapy within the past 12 months.
    - Following an attack of severe colitis.
- Surgery:
  - May be required:
    - As an emergency therapy during an acute severe attack of UC for perforation, toxic dilatation, haemorrhage etc.
    - If an acute flare-up is not settled by medical therapy.
    - In patients who experience frequent relapses, or in whom surgery would restore quality of life.
  - Options include:
    - Colectomy with permanent ileostomy.
    - Construction of an ileoanal 'pouch' which restores intestinal continuity and avoids a stoma.
  - Patients should undergo careful counselling prior to such surgery.

COMPLICATIONS

- Colonic complications:
  - Toxic megacolon.
  - Bowel perforation.
  - Colorectal cancer.
- Opportunistic infections (due to immunosuppressive medications).

8.6 DIVERTICULAR DISEASE

DEFINITION

- Diverticulae: out-pouching of the colonic mucosa/submucosa through a weakened area of the colonic wall.
- The presence of multiple diverticulae is referred to as diverticulosis/diverticular disease (see Figure 8.3).
- Diverticulitis refers to the inflammation of one or more of these diverticula with associated abdominal pain, altered bowel habit, bloating and/or fever.

EPIDEMIOLOGY

- Affects 5–10% of the population over the age of 45 years, and 80% of those older than 85 years in Western society.
- Male predominance is present before the age of 50 years with equal gender distribution after the age of 60.
- Diverticulosis is most common in the sigmoid colon.

AETIOLOGY/RISK FACTORS

- High luminal pressure causes mucosal protrusion through areas of weakness in the muscularis propria where the vasa rectae penetrate the bowel wall, causing the diverticulae.

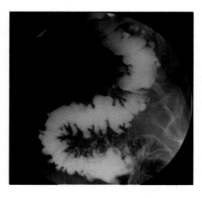

Figure 8.3 Barium enema image showing diverticular disease.

- Dietary risk factors:
  - High intake of carbohydrates and red meat.
  - Low fibre intake.
- Other aetiological risk factors:
  - Altered colonic microbial flora.
  - NSAIDs (through decreased prostaglandin synthesis which impairs the colonic mucosal barrier).

CLINICAL FEATURES

- Usually asymptomatic unless the diverticulae become inflamed leading to diverticulitis.
- History:
  - Rectal bleeding (haematochezia).
  - Abdominal pain.
  - Fever.
  - Nausea and vomiting.
  - Dysuria: frequency, urgency.
  - Constipation/diarrhoea.
- Examination:
  - Localized tenderness (usually localized to the left iliac fossa).
  - Tender mass – may indicate abscess formation.
  - Diffuse abdominal tenderness and guarding – may suggest free perforation or purulent peritonitis.
  - Hypoactive bowel sounds.
  - Haemodynamic instability (if there is free perforation).

INVESTIGATIONS

- Blood tests:
  - FBC: leucocytosis.
  - ESR/CRP: raised inflammatory markers.
- Imaging:
  - Erect CXR/AXR if there are features of obstruction/perforation:
    - Bowel dilatation, air-fluid level, air under the diaphragm.
  - Barium enema.
  - CT abdomen.
  - Colonoscopy – performed 8 weeks following an acute episode to exclude malignancy.

MANAGEMENT

- Bowel rest/clear fluid diet.
- Pharmacological intervention:
  - Antibiotic therapy to cover for infections: augmentin/cefuroxime and metronidazole.

Gastroenterology

- Hospitalization is usually required in the following circumstances:
  - Elderly patient.
  - Immunosuppressed patient.
  - Signs of systemic infection.
  - Multiple comorbidities.

COMPLICATIONS

- Acute diverticulitis.
- Pericolic or pelvic abscess.
- Purulent or faeculent peritonitis.
- Fistula to adjacent organs.
- Bowel obstruction.
- Diverticular haemorrhage.

8.7 ISCHAEMIC COLITIS

DEFINITION

- Necrosis of a segment of bowel wall due to insufficient blood supply.
- May present as an occlusive or non-occlusive form.
- Severity may vary between superficial mucosal injury and full thickness bowel wall necrosis leading to acute gangrenous colitis.
- Usually results in self-limiting injury to the colon.

EPIDEMIOLOGY

- The splenic flexure, descending colon and sigmoid are most commonly affected.
- Approximately 90% of cases occur in patients over the age of 60 years.

AETIOLOGY

- Mesenteric venous thrombosis/arterial thrombosis.
- Embolic events (arterial, cholesterol, infective).

RISK FACTORS

- Hypoperfusion states:
  - Congestive heart failure.
  - Hypotension.
  - Cardiopulmonary bypass.
  - Aorto-iliac reconstruction surgery.
  - Dehydration.
  - Shock (due to various causes).
- Mechanical colonic obstruction: volvulus, tumours, adhesions etc.
- Medications: antibiotics (penicillin derivatives), diuretics, NSAIDs, oestrogens etc.

- Hypercoagulability states:
  - Factor V Leiden (FVL) mutations.
  - Protein C, protein S and antithrombin III deficiencies.
  - Antiphospholipid antibody syndrome.
- Vasculitides:
  - SLE.
  - Polyarteritis nodosa.
  - Rheumatoid vasculitis.
- Other:
  - Sickle cell disease.
  - Smoking.
  - Colonic infections causing haemorrhagic colitis.
  - Cholesterol emboli.

CLINICAL FEATURES

- Diagnosis requires a high index of clinical suspicion.
- History:
  - Sudden onset of crampy lower abdominal pain (usually left iliac fossa).
  - Rectal bleeding/bloody diarrhoea.
- Examination:
  - May be normal in mild cases.
  - Increasing abdominal tenderness and guarding with a temperature suggest full thickness infarction and peritonitis.
  - Peritoneal signs (if there is perforation or peritonitis).

DIFFERENTIAL DIAGNOSIS

- Infectious colitis.
- IBD.
- Diverticulitis.
- Colonic carcinoma.

INVESTIGATIONS

- Stool cultures – exclude bacterial causes of haemorrhagic colitis.
- Imaging:
  - AXR:
    - Thumb-printing, air-filled loops, mural thickening.
  - Barium enema (uncommonly used):
    - Thumb-printing, ridges, ulcers, oedema, mural deformity, strictures.
  - Flexible sigmoidoscopy/colonoscopy:
    - Segmental petechial bleeding, pale mucosa, haemorrhagic ulcers.
    - In severe cases, colonoscopy is contraindicated due to the risk of perforation.

Gastroenterology

- Abdominal CT:
  - Wall thickening, pericolic fat stranding, mucosal and submucosal haemorrhage.
- Angiography (rarely necessary):
  - If acute mesenteric ischaemia is considered.
- Colonic biopsy.

- Acute management:
  - Diet:
    - Bowel rest with intravenous fluid administration:
      - Very mild cases may be treated with liquid diet.
    - Parenteral nutrition may be required during prolonged illness.
  - Pharmacological intervention:
    - Broad-spectrum IV antibiotics.
    - Withdrawal of possible causative medications.
  - Rectal and NG tubes – in patients with marked colonic distension.
  - Surgery (rarely required).

- Accounts for <5% of intestinal ischaemic disease.
- Usually caused by atherosclerosis.
- Usually presents with abdominal pain within 30 minutes of eating, resolving over 1–3 hours.
- Investigations:
  - Doppler ultrasound, MRA, angiography.
- Management:
  - Angioplasty/stent.
  - Surgical revascularization.

8.8 SOLITARY RECTAL ULCER SYNDROME

- Uncommon traumatic lesion of the anterior rectal wall caused by straining due to functional disorders of defaecation.
- Mucosal prolapse is the most common underlying mechanism in solitary rectal ulcer syndrome (SURS).
- Lesions may be multiple despite the name of the condition.

EPIDEMIOLOGY

- Usually seen in young adults:
  - Most commonly in the third decade in men.
  - Most commonly in the fourth decade in women.

CLINICAL FEATURES

- History:
  - Rectal bleeding.
  - Passage of mucus.
  - Straining during defaecation.
  - Feeling of incomplete evacuation.
  - Abnormal bowel habit.

INVESTIGATIONS

- A diagnosis of SRUS is based upon symptomatology in combination with histological and endoscopic findings.
- Endoscopy:
  - Appearances are very variable and may include hyperaemic mucosa, small or giant ulcers or polypoid lesions.
- Pathognomonic histological findings include:
  - Mucosal thickening.
  - Elongation/distortion of glands.
  - Fibrosis.
  - Extension of smooth muscle fibres between crypts.
- Defecography:
  - Sometimes useful for identifying internal/external mucosal prolapse.
- Endorectal ultrasound:
  - Shows thickening of muscularis propria.

DIFFERENTIAL DIAGNOSIS

- IBD.
- Infectious cause: amoebiasis, lymphogranuloma venereum, secondary syphilis.
- Malignancy.
- Trauma (e.g. stercoral ulceration).
- Medication effect: nicorandil, ergotamine tartrate-containing suppositories.

MANAGEMENT

- Patient education and behavioural modifications including defaecation training:
  - Increased fibre intake.
  - Avoidance of straining and anal digitation.

Gastroenterology

- Biofeedback: aim to reduce excessive straining with defaecation by correcting abnormal pelvic floor behaviour.
- Pharmacological intervention:
  - Use of bulk laxatives.
  - Topical treatments: sucralfate enema, fibrin glue.
- Surgery:
  - Considered if there is evidence of internal/external prolapse.

8.9 PSEUDOMEMBRANOUS COLITIS

DEFINITION

- An infectious colitis caused by *C. difficile* bacterium (gram-positive rod) (see Figure 8.4).

EPIDEMIOLOGY

- *C. difficile* is present in the gut of up to 3% of adults and 66% of children, but rarely causes active infection in children or healthy adults.
- The bacteria may colonize up to 40% of hospitalized patients.
- Over 80% of *C. difficile* diarrhoea is seen in patients over the age of 65 years.

PATHOPHYSIOLOGY

- *C. difficile* is a gram-positive, anaerobic, toxigenic, spore-forming rod:
  - *C. difficile* spores are heat and alcohol resistant.

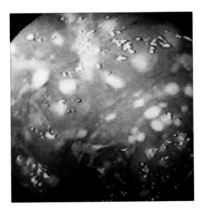

Figure 8.4 Colonoscopy image showing pseudomembranous colitis from a patient with *Clostridium difficile* infection.

- The bacteria produce two toxins which cause the disease:
  - Toxin A: an inflammatory endotoxin that increases mucosal permeability.
  - Toxin B: a cytotoxin.

MICRO-facts

It is important to remember that alcohol gel is not effective against *Clostridium difficile* spores; thorough and regular hand washing with soap and water is an essential preventive strategy against spread of *C. difficile* bacteria.

RISK FACTORS

- PPI therapy.
- IBD.
- Old age.
- Use of broad-spectrum antibiotics.
- Multiple comorbidities.

PREVENTION

- Cautious use of antibiotics.
- Routine hand washing by hospital personnel with soap and water before and after patient contact.
- Use of gloves and apron during contact with infected patients.
- Isolation of suspected cases.
- Treatment of asymptomatic *C. difficile* carriers is not recommended as it may prolong the carrier state.

CLINICAL FEATURES

- History:
  - Diarrhoea (watery or mucoid).
  - Dehydration.
  - Nausea and vomiting.
  - Fever.
  - Abdominal pain.

INVESTIGATION

- Stool culture for detection of *C. difficile* antigen and/or toxin in symptomatic patients:
  - Should be sent as soon as *C. difficile* infection is suspected.

Gastroenterology

> # MICRO-facts
>
> Current available tests for the detection of *Clostridium difficile* include:
> - Toxin enzyme immunoassay (EIA) tests: detect the presence of *C. difficile* toxin(s).
> - Toxin gene tests (NAAT or PCR): detect the presence of toxin gene(s).
> - Glutamate dehydrogenase (GDH) EIA: detects an antigen that is produced in high amounts by *C. difficile*.
> - Cytotoxin and cytotoxigenic culture: the most sensitive tests although not commonly used due to cost and turnaround time.

DIFFERENTIAL DIAGNOSIS

- Other causes of acute bacterial diarrhoea (campylobacter infections, salmonellosis etc.).
- Acute viral gastroenteritis (e.g. norovirus).
- Parasitic diarrhoea (e.g. amoebiasis).
- Inflammatory causes (e.g. IBD, microscopic colitis, diverticulitis).
- Ischaemic colitis.
- Drug-induced diarrhoea.
- Overflow diarrhoea.
- IBS.

MANAGEMENT

- Stop existing antibiotics, PPIs and gut motility drugs if possible.
- Patient isolation: should ideally be undertaken within 2 hours of diarrhoea onset.
- Fluid replacement.
- Antibiotics:
  - Oral metronidazole (first-line therapy).
  - Oral vancomycin (should be considered if there is no response to metronidazole after 2–3 days).
  - IV metronidazole for patients who cannot tolerate oral antibiotics or antibiotics via NG tube.
- Other pharmacological interventions:
  - Oral probiotics (e.g. lactobacillus GG): shown to be effective in preventing relapse.
  - Faecal enema from healthy individuals.
- Surgery:
  - Diverting ileostomy or colectomy in severe cases or for complications.

COMPLICATIONS

- Toxic megacolon.
- Bowel perforation.
- Recurrence:
  - Occurs in up to 30% of cases.
  - Management is as for an acute attack.

8.10 COLORECTAL CANCER

EPIDEMIOLOGY

- Second most common cause of cancer death in Western Europe.
- Fourth most common cancer in the UK.
- Incidence increases sharply from 50 years with the highest incidence in patients over 85 years of age.
- Over 95% of cases of colorectal cancer (CRC) are adenocarcinomas; other less common tumours include lymphoma, leiomyosarcomas and carcinoid tumours.
- Approximately 25% of patients with CRC have a family history of the disease.

RISK FACTORS

- Family history of CRC:
  - Inherited (autosomal dominant) syndromes:
    - Non-polyposis syndromes (more common):
      - Hereditary non-polyposis CRC (HNPCC): 40% lifetime risk of developing CRC due to mutations in DNA mismatch repair genes.
    - Polyposis syndromes (less common):
      - Familial adenomatous polyposis (FAP): diffuse colorectal polyposis with 100% risk of developing CRC by the age of 40 years due to mutation of the APC gene.
      - Turcot's syndrome: colonic polyposis and CNS tumours due to mutations of the APC gene or DNA mismatch repair genes.
      - Peutz–Jeghers syndrome: multiple hamartomatous polyps throughout the GI tract due to mutations of STK11/LKB1.
- IBD (extensive UC or Crohn's colitis).
- Previous CRC.
- Smoking.
- Obesity.
- Dietary factors (low fibre intake, high red meat intake etc.).
- Diabetes mellitus and acromegaly (insulin-like growth hormone is a growth factor for colonic mucosal cells).

Gastroenterology

PATHOPHYSIOLOGY

- The majority of CRCs follow a stepwise chronological sequence of molecular and genetic changes leading to a transformation from normal epithelium to overt malignancy.
- This is depicted in the following diagram:
  Normal epithelium → (Mutation of APC gene) → Hyperproliferative epithelium → (K-RAS mutation) → Early adenoma → Intermediate adenoma → Late adenoma → (Loss of p53) → Carcinoma → Metastasis

> **MICRO-reference**
> For further information on the pathophysiology of colorectal cancers, see: Fearon ER, Vogelstein B. A genetic model for colorectal tumorigenesis. Cell 1990; 61:759–767.

CLINICAL FEATURES

- History:
  - Vague abdominal pain.
  - Fatigue.
  - Weight loss.
  - Rectal bleeding.
  - Altered bowel habit (usually to more frequent or looser stools).
  - Haematochezia: the passage of fresh red blood PR.
- Examination:
  - Acute abdomen (due to intestinal obstruction or perforation).
  - Palpable abdominal mass (including liver or rectal mass).
  - Lymphadenopathy.
  - Anaemia.

INVESTIGATIONS

- Digital rectal examination: for suspected rectal cancers.
- Serological investigations:
  - FBC, U&E, LFTs.
  - Carcinoembryonic antigen (CEA) – not a diagnostic test but useful for monitoring for recurrence.
- Colonoscopy with biopsy:
  - Alternative imaging methods include barium enema or CT colonography.
- Grading/staging of tumours:
  - CT staging: chest, abdomen, pelvis (see Figure 8.5).
  - MRI pelvis for rectal tumours.

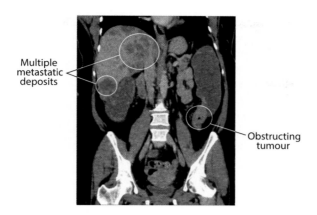

Figure 8.5 Computed tomography (CT) scan showing an obstructing colorectal carcinoma in the descending colon and metastatic deposits in the liver.

MICRO-reference

For full NICE guidance on methods of staging of colorectal cancer including TNM classification, see: http://pathways.nice.org.uk/pathways/colorectal-cancer/staging-colorectal-cancer

---

SCREENING

- National bowel cancer screening programme in the UK:
  - Offers screening every 2 years to all men and women aged 60–74 years:
    - Initial screening is done using faecal occult blood (FOB) testing:
      - If positive, subsequent colonoscopy is offered.
  - Flexible sigmoidoscopy offered to all patients at age 55 (currently being rolled out in England).

MANAGEMENT

- Surgical intervention:
  - Curative surgery is the preferred option in a patient with no distant metastasis or prohibitive comorbid conditions.
- Chemotherapy: 5-fluorouracil (5FU-based regimes) used as neoadjuvant therapy for advanced disease or for palliative therapy.
- Radiotherapy:
  - Used in patients with node-positive disease or trans-mural rectal cancer.
  - Used as palliative therapy in bone or brain metastasis.

- Palliative interventions:
  - Colonic stenting to treat acute obstruction prior to surgery or for palliation of obstructive symptoms.
- Follow-up management:
  - Colonoscopy every 5 years.
  - CT within 2 years.
  - CEA every 6 months for 3 years.

COMPLICATIONS

- Bowel obstruction.
- Perforation.
- Recurrence of CRC.

PROGNOSIS

- Overall 5-year survival of approximately 64%.

MICRO-case

A 24-year-old normally fit and well PhD student attends his GP with gradually worsening diarrhoea over the last 5 weeks. He had been to the GP 3 weeks ago; a stool MC&S was negative. He is now having lower abdominal pain prior to defaecation and is feeling very washed out to the point where he can no longer carry on with his PhD project. He is especially concerned about his increased bowel frequency, approximately seven times per day and at least twice at nighttime. He is having blood mixed with loose stools almost on every bowel movement during the past week. He has lost 5 kg in weight. His last holiday abroad was 2 years ago to mainland Spain. He is a non-smoker and he is not on any regular medications.

On examination, he looks pale. Vital signs are as follows: BP 115/82 mmHg, P 80 bpm, RR 14 breaths per minute, T 37.9°C, O_2 sat. 99%. He has lower abdominal tenderness, but no rebound or guarding is apparent. Bowel sounds are normal.

The GP decides to admit him to the acute medical unit at the local hospital that same day. He is seen by the junior admitting doctor who decides on the following investigations:

- FBC, U&Es, CRP, ESR, LFTs.
- Stool culture×3 including *Clostridium difficile* toxin (CDT).
- AXR.
- Blood culture.

Significant blood results are: Hb: 101 g/L; MCV: 80 fL; WCC: 9.1×10^9/L; Platelets: 415×10^9/L; CRP: 52 mg/L; ESR: 35 mm/h. AXR reveals a degree of mucosal thickening on the left side of the colon.

continued...

continued...

Following discussion with the senior medical physician, he is treated as a new diagnosis of acute severe ulcerative colitis. He is started on IV hydrocortisone 100 mg QDS, IV fluid and prophylactic low-molecular-weight heparin. The diagnosis is supported by findings of friable colonic mucosa with spontaneous bleeding ahead of the scope and superficial ulceration on flexible sigmoidoscopy examination the following day.

His bowel frequency reduces to four times a day after 2 days and he no longer has lower abdominal tenderness. Repeat blood markers show CRP: 11 mg/L; ESR: 21 mm/h; WCC: 11.2×10^9/L; Hb: 105 g/L; and Platelets: 350×10^9/L. Stool cultures remain negative. IV hydrocortisone is switched to oral prednisolone on day 5 and he is successfully discharged the following day.

Key points:

- Prophylactic low-molecular-weight heparin should be considered for all patients with severe ulcerative colitis due to the high risk of thromboembolic events.
- Stool culture to exclude acute bacterial colitis including *C. difficile*-associated diarrhoea is necessary due to increased incidence of infective colitis in inflammatory bowel disease.
- Close daily monitoring should be carried out with particular attention to the patient's vital signs, bowel frequency, abdominal examination and laboratory markers (U&Es, CRP, FBC, ESR).
- Travis criteria: On day 3 of corticosteroid therapy, if CRP >45 mg/L with stool frequency of 3–8 times/24 hr or if bowel frequency remains more than 8 times/24 hr, urgent surgical assessment should be sought and further step-up medical (ciclosporin or infliximab therapy) or surgical (subtotal colectomy and end ileostomy) intervention should be considered.

MICRO-references
Travis SP, Farrant JM, Ricketts C, et al. Predicting outcome in severe ulcerative colitis. *Gut* 1996; 38: 905–910.
    For further information on the pathophysiology of colorectal cancers, see: Fearon ER, Vogelstein B. A genetic model for colorectal tumorigenesis. *Cell* 1990; 61: 759–767.

9 Pancreatobiliary disease

9.1 ANATOMY

ANATOMY OF THE PANCREAS

- The pancreas is both an endocrine and an exocrine organ.
- It may be split into four anatomical regions: head, neck, body and tail (see Figure 9.1).
- The main pancreatic duct joins together with the common bile duct to enter the second part of the duodenum at the ampulla of Vater:
  - This allows for transfer of pancreatic enzymes and bile into the small intestine.
- The superior and inferior pancreaticoduodenal arteries, as well as the splenic artery, supply the pancreas with blood.

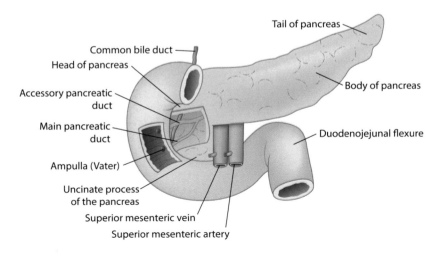

Figure 9.1 Anatomical diagram of pancreas.

ANATOMY OF THE BILIARY TRACT

- The hepatocytes of the liver secrete bile into the bile canaliculi, which merge to form bile ducts.
- These bile ducts anastomose to form progressively wider ducts, which eventually form the left and right hepatic ducts.
- These merge to produce the common hepatic duct.
- Bile is transferred from the gallbladder via the cystic duct, which joins the common hepatic duct to form the common bile duct.
- The common bile duct joins the main pancreatic duct and opens at the ampulla of Vater.
- The gallbladder may be divided into three anatomical regions: fundus, body and neck.
- The gallbladder acts as a site of storage for the body's bile.

9.2 PHYSIOLOGY

PHYSIOLOGY OF THE PANCREAS

- The pancreas secretes a number of digestive enzymes (see Figure 9.2).
- The proteolytic enzymes secreted by the pancreas are stored in their inactive form to prevent damage to pancreatic tissue:
  - They are activated in the duodenum by the action of intestinal enzymes:
    - Enterokinases from the brush border convert trypsinogen to trypsin.
    - Trypsin, in turn, activates further trypsinogen as well as other endopeptidases.
- The endocrine function of the pancreas comprises discrete clusters of cells known as the islets of Langerhans:
  - The main cells types are α-cells secreting glucagon, β-cells secreting insulin, δ-cells secreting somatostatin and PP cells secreting pancreatic polypeptide.

PHYSIOLOGY OF BILIARY SECRETION

- Bile contains a number of substances. These include:
  - Water, bile salts, bicarbonate ions, cholesterol, bile pigments, lecithin, conjugated bilirubin.
- Secretion of bile is stimulated by cholecystokinin (CCK), which causes contraction of the gallbladder and relaxation of the sphincter of Oddi:
  - CCK is secreted in response to the presence of fat in the duodenum.
  - Bile secretion is inhibited by the action of somatostatin.

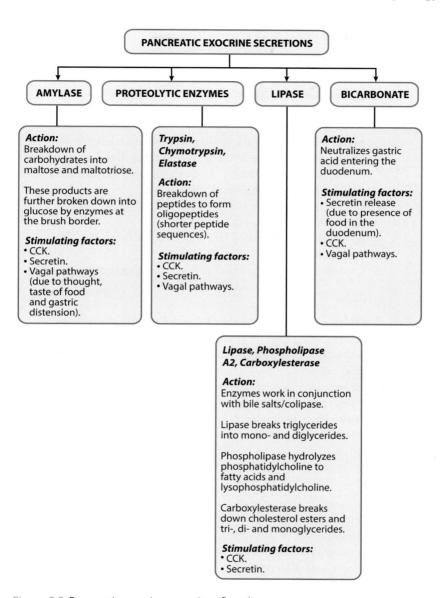

Figure 9.2 Pancreatic exocrine secretions flow diagram.

- The main functions of bile include:
  - Emulsification of fats (breaking fats down into smaller droplets to increase the surface area over which pancreatic lipase can work).
  - Neutralizes gastric acid (contains bicarbonate ions).

9.3 CHOLELITHIASIS

DEFINITION

- More commonly known as 'gallstones'.
- Types of gallstone include:
  - Cholesterol stones:
    - Account for 80% of gallstones in Western countries.
    - Often due to excessive levels of cholesterol in the bile:
      - Associated with cholesterol supersaturation, decreased bile acid synthesis and gallbladder hypomotility.
  - Bile pigment stones:
    - Generally composed of calcium salts.
    - Associated with increased rate of haemolysis.
  - Mixed stones:
    - Contain cholesterol, calcium salts and bile pigment.

RISK FACTORS

- Female gender: oestrogens increased cholesterol secretion into the bile.
- Older age.
- Obesity: increased cholesterol synthesis and secretion into the bile.
- Diabetes mellitus.
- Pregnancy: increased cholesterol secretion into the bile.
- Family history: patients with a first-degree relative with gallstones are 4.5 times more likely to develop gallstones.
- Terminal ileal disease due to loss of bile salts (e.g. Crohn's disease).

CLINICAL FEATURES

- History:
  - Most cases are asymptomatic (may be an incidental finding on imaging).
  - Abdominal pain (biliary colic):
    - Usually localized to the epigastrium or right upper quadrant.
    - Severe pain associated with ingestion of fatty foods.
    - Pain may radiate to the back or the right shoulder tip.
    - Pain lasting for >6 hours may be suggestive of cholecystitis or pancreatitis.
  - Nausea and vomiting.
- Examination:
  - Clinical jaundice: obstruction of the bile duct causes a conjugated hyperbilirubinaemia.

Gastroenterology

- Abdominal tenderness:
  - Pain in the right upper quadrant.
  - Murphy's sign positive:
    - Pain is elicited when pressure is applied to the right upper quadrant during inspiration.

INVESTIGATIONS

- Bloods:
  - FBC: raised WCC may indicate acute cholecystitis/cholangitis.
  - LFTs: may show evidence of obstructive jaundice (if the common bile duct is obstructed).
- Plain abdominal radiograph (abdominal X-ray [AXR]):
  - Only 10% of stones are radio-opaque and visible on AXR.
- Abdominal ultrasound scan:
  - Demonstrates gallstones >2 mm in the gallbladder in 95% of cases.
  - Only demonstrates 50% of gallstones in the bile duct.
- Magnetic retrograde cholangiopancreatography (MRCP):
  - Demonstrates approximately 95% of stones.
- CT scan:
  - Only demonstrates calcified stones: main indication is to detect complications.
- Endoscopic ultrasound (EUS):
  - Most accurate investigation for bile duct stones.
- ERCP (endoscopic retrograde cholangiopancreatography):
  - Used to remove diagnosed bile duct stones. No longer used as a diagnostic procedure owing to associated risks.

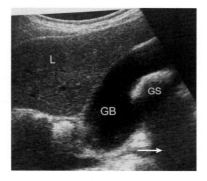

Figure 9.3 Ultrasound image of the gallbladder and liver.

MANAGEMENT

- Pharmacological intervention:
    - If the patient is asymptomatic (incidental finding) no treatment is required.
    - Analgesia (for biliary colic).
    - Extracorporeal shock wave lithotripsy (rarely used):
        - Use of high-pressure sound waves to fragment the gallstone.
        - Indicated in patients with a non-obstructed, functional gallbladder with non-calcified gallstones less than 20 mm in diameter.
- Surgical management:
    - Laparoscopic cholecystectomy: management of choice for symptomatic gallstones.
    - ERCP: management of bile duct stones.

COMPLICATIONS

- Cholecystitis (see MICRO-facts box):
    - Inflammation of the gallbladder is usually due to a stone becoming impacted in the cystic duct.
    - Presentation is with acute abdominal pain, which may radiate to the back or to the right shoulder tip and fever.
- Cholangitis (see MICRO-facts box):
    - Infection of the biliary tract secondary to obstruction of the bile duct by gallstones (occasionally obstruction is caused by a tumour).
    - Presentation is with fever, severe abdominal pain and jaundice.
- Pancreatitis.
- Gallstone ileus:
    - Formation of a fistula from the gallbladder to the duodenum secondary to chronic inflammation.

MICRO-facts

Table illustrating the different pathological presentations of gallstones and acute pancreatitis:

	DEFINITION	CLINICAL FEATURES	INVESTIGATIONS	MANAGEMENT
Biliary colic	Pain caused by impacted gallstone at the site of the cystic duct or ampulla of Vater.	• Colicky pain in the right hypochondrium, radiating to the shoulder. • Vomiting.	• Largely a clinical diagnosis made on the basis of clinical features. • USS shows gallbladder stones, may show dilated CBD or bile duct stones. • LFTs may show obstructive picture (if gallstone is impacted). • MRCP to be considered if LFTs are deranged or bile duct is dilated on USS.	• Analgesia (may require morphine). • ERCP for bile duct stone. • Cholecystectomy/surgical exploration of the bile duct.
Acute cholecystitis	Generally caused by impacted gallstone at the gallbladder neck causing outflow obstruction and leading to inflammation.	• Colicky pain in the right hypochondrium. • Fever. • Localized peritonism. • Murphy's sign positive (see Section 9.3).	• Raised WCC. • USS shows thickening of the gallbladder wall and gallstones. • Abdominal X-ray may show calcified stones.	• Analgesia. • IV fluids. • IV antibiotics (if there is evidence of sepsis): (metronidazole + cefuroxime/co-amoxiclav). • Cholecystectomy.

continued...

Gastroenterology

continued...

	DEFINITION	CLINICAL FEATURES	INVESTIGATIONS	MANAGEMENT
Ascending cholangitis	Biliary tract inflammation and infection caused by stasis of bile due to blockage of the CBD by gallstones.	Charcot's triad: • Colicky pain in the right hypochondrium. • Fever. • Jaundice.	• Raised WCC. • Raised CRP. • LFTs show an obstructive pattern. • USS may show dilatation of the CBD or stones. • Blood cultures. • MRCP if bile duct stone is not visualized on USS.	• Analgesia. • IV fluids and resuscitation as required. • IV antibiotics (cefuroxime and metronidazole/co-amoxiclav). • ERCP.
Acute pancreatitis	Obstruction of the pancreatic duct/bile duct by CBD stone.	• Epigastric/upper abdominal pain. • Nausea and vomiting. • Epigastric tenderness.	• Serum amylase/lipase. • WCC. • CRP. • USS shows swollen pancreas, dilated CBD. • CT scan shows peri-pancreatic collections. • MRCP if CBD stone is suspected.	• Analgesia. • NBM initially. • IV fluids. • Antibiotics for severe cases (use Glasgow score to determine). • ERCP if CBD stone is present.

CBD, common bile duct; CRP, C-reactive protein; ERCP, endoscopic retrograde cholangiopancreatography; IV, intravenous; LFT, liver function test; MRCP, magnetic resonance cholangiopancreatography; NBM, nil by mouth; USS, ultrasound scan; WCC, white cell count.

9.4 GALLBLADDER CARCINOMA

EPIDEMIOLOGY

- Incidence of 2.5 in 100,000.
- Approximately 85% are adenocarcinomas.
- Other types include:
  - Squamous cell carcinoma.
  - Small cell carcinoma.
  - Sarcoma.
  - Neuroendocrine tumours.
- Generally occur in patients over the age of 60 years.
- Three times more common in women.

RISK FACTORS

- Gallstones:
  - Up to 90% of patients with gallbladder carcinoma have gallstones:
    - However, only 0.5% of patients with gallstones will develop gallbladder cancer.
- Chronic cholecystitis (inflammation of the gallbladder):
  - Causes 'porcelain gallbladder' due to formation of calcium deposits.
- Obesity.

CLINICAL FEATURES

- Carcinoma of the gallbladder is often found during routine investigation of suspected gallstones.
- History:
  - Abdominal pain.
  - Fever.
  - Weight loss.
  - Anorexia.
  - Jaundice.
- Examination:
  - Abdominal mass: right hypochondrium.
  - Virchow's node (see Section 6.7).
  - Jaundice.
  - Tenderness on palpation.

Gastroenterology

> ## MICRO-facts
> Courvoisier's sign:
> - An enlarged gallbladder present in a jaundiced patient:
>   - Likely to be due to carcinoma of the head of the pancreas.
>   - Not commonly seen in a patient with gallstones, as this causes fibrosis, and not enlargement of the gallbladder.

INVESTIGATIONS

- Bloods:
  - LFTs: may show raised ALP, γGT (usually following obstruction of the bile duct and the development of jaundice or due to local infiltration of the liver).
  - CA 19-9 tumour marker:
    - Levels will be elevated in patients with pancreatic, colorectal, hepatobiliary and gallbladder carcinoma.
- Ultrasound scan.
- CT scan.
- MRI/MRCP.
- EUS.
- Laparoscopy: some cancers can be found incidentally at laparoscopy.

MANAGEMENT

- Surgical intervention:
  - Cholecystectomy:
    - T2 or T3 cancers require cholecystectomy with the removal of a portion of the adjacent liver and lymph nodes.
    - T4 cancers have a poor prognosis even with extensive resection.
    - May be curative in early-stage disease.
- Adjuvant treatment:
  - Chemotherapy: 5-FU regimens have a 5–30% response rate.
  - Radiotherapy: used to control microscopic residual foci or palliation.

PROGNOSIS

- Most patients with gallbladder carcinoma present late, and the prognosis is therefore generally poor:
  - Only 10–20% of patients presenting with gallbladder carcinoma have early-stage disease (confined to the gallbladder wall) with a 95–98% survival.
  - Patients with advanced disease show a 5-year survival rate of 2–4%.

9.5 CHOLANGIOCARCINOMA

DEFINITION

- Carcinoma arising from biliary epithelium: may be intrahepatic or extrahepatic.

EPIDEMIOLOGY

- Incidence of 1–2 cases per 100,000.
- Over 90% are adenocarcinomas:
  - A small minority are squamous cell carcinomas.
- Cholangiocarcinoma has a higher incidence in Southeast Asia secondary to chronic infection of the biliary system by *Clonorchis sinensis* (liver fluke).
- The Bismuth-Corlette classification of location of tumour is used in the staging of hilar cholangiocarcinoma (see MICRO-reference box).

> **MICRO-reference**
> For more information on the Bismuth-Corlette classification of hilar cholangiocarcinoma, see: http://radiopaedia.org/articles/bismuth-corlette-classification

RISK FACTORS

- Primary sclerosing cholangitis.
- Intrahepatic stones.
- Congenital abnormalities of the biliary tract (e.g. choledochal cysts).
- Liver fluke (*Cl. sinensis*):
  - Contracted through ingestion of infected fish.
  - Common cause of cholangiocarcinoma in Southeast Asia.

CLINICAL FEATURES

- Generally shows a local pattern of spread with liver metastases.
- History:
  - 90% present with jaundice.
  - Abdominal pain.
  - Pale stools: obstructive picture.
  - Pruritis.
  - Fever.
  - Weight loss.
- Examination:
  - Jaundice.
  - Tenderness in the right hypochondrium: may radiate to the back.

- Palpable mass: right hypochondrium.
- Hepatomegaly.

INVESTIGATIONS

- Bloods:
  - FBC: rule out complications (e.g. cholangitis).
  - LFTs: usually show a cholestatic picture (see Chapter 4).
  - Tumour markers CA 19-9 and CEA (these are non-specific).
- Abdominal ultrasound scan.
- CT scan.
- MRCP.
- EUS ± biopsy for distal lesions.
- ERCP ± brushing (allows cytological confirmation of cause of biliary stricture in many cases) and also allows stenting.

MANAGEMENT

- Surgical resection:
  - May include partial hepatectomy for intrahepatic or perihilar lesions depending upon the stage of the disease.
  - Pancreaticoduodenectomy (Whipple's procedure) is performed for distal tumours.
  - Adjuvant radiotherapy/chemotherapy is not routinely used.
- Palliative procedures:
  - Biliary drainage:
    - Insertion of one or more stents into the biliary tree via ERCP or percutaneous transhepatic cholangiography.
    - Biliary-enteric bypass.
  - Chemotherapy: gemcitabine and cisplatin in combination is recommended for unresectable disease.
  - External beam radiotherapy: is not used routinely but may be of benefit for local metastases or uncontrolled bleeding.

PROGNOSIS

- Less than one-third of patients will benefit from surgical resection at presentation.
- Patients who undergo surgical resection with curative intent show a 5-year survival rate of approximately 40%.

9.6 ACUTE PANCREATITIS

DEFINITION

- Rapid onset of inflammation of the pancreas.

AETIOLOGY

- 'GET SMASHED' causes (see MICRO-facts box).
- Other causes include:
  - Cystic fibrosis.
  - Viral infection (e.g. Coxsackie virus).
  - Hereditary (mutations of the cationic trypsinogen gene, PRSS1).

MICRO-facts

'GET SMASHED' mnemonic for causes of pancreatitis:

- G – Gallstones (most common cause)
- E – Ethanol (alcohol is a common cause in the Western world)
- T – Trauma
- S – Steroids
- M – Mumps
- A – Autoimmune
- S – Scorpion sting
- H – Hyperlipidaemia, hypercalcaemia
- E – ERCP (procedure may cause trauma to the pancreas)
- D – Drugs: corticosteroids, thiazide diuretics, sulfonamides etc.

PATHOPHYSIOLOGY

- Pancreatitis occurs when the pancreatic enzymes are activated prematurely causing destruction of pancreatic tissue:
  - In chronic pancreatitis, normal tissue is replaced by fibrosis causing irreversible damage (see Section 9.7).

CLINICAL FEATURES

- History:
  - Abdominal pain:
    - Severe epigastric pain, which may radiate to the back.
    - Exacerbated by eating and eased by sitting forwards.
  - Nausea and vomiting.
- Examination:
  - Fever.
  - Jaundice:
    - Suggestive of bile duct stones.
    - May also be due to compression of the bile duct by an oedematous pancreatic head.
  - Cullen's sign:
    - Periumbilical bruising due to extravasation of haemorrhagic pancreatic exudate associated with pancreatic necrosis.

Gastroenterology

- Grey Turner's sign:
  - Bruising of the flank regions due to extravasation of haemorrhagic pancreatic exudate associated with pancreatic necrosis.
- Signs of shock in severe cases: tachycardia, hypotension etc.

INVESTIGATIONS

- Blood tests:
  - Serum amylase:
    - Raised in pancreatitis (>1000 units/mL considered diagnostic).
    - Increases within 6–12 hours of onset, and is cleared rapidly from the blood (half-life of 10 hours).
  - Serum lipase:
    - Raised levels are more specific for pancreatitis than serum amylase (since almost all of the body's lipase is produced by the pancreas).
    - Remains elevated for a longer period than serum amylase.
  - FBC: raised WCC due to underlying inflammation/rarely infection.
  - LFTs: raised due to inflammatory process/duct obstruction.
  - Glucose: raised levels may signify damage to the insulin-secreting β-cells of the pancreas.
- AXR:
  - May show underlying aetiology (gallstones etc.).
- Abdominal ultrasound scan: shows pseudocysts, gallstones, bile ducts.
- CT scan: shows pseudocysts, pancreatic necrosis.
- MRCP: demonstrates common bile duct stones not seen on ultrasound.
- EUS: used to demonstrate bile duct stones not visualized by other methods.

MANAGEMENT

- Supportive treatment:
  - IV fluids (patient must be kept nil-by-mouth).
  - Patient may require enteral nutrition (usually nasojejunal).
  - Analgesia/antiemetics.
  - IV antibiotics: given as prophylaxis in severe cases.
- Management of the underlying condition, e.g. removal of bile duct stones.
- Surgery:
  - Indicated if the patient suffers from infected pancreatic necrosis.
  - Generally consists of surgical debridement of necrotic tissue.

COMPLICATIONS

- Infection:
  - May complicate pancreatic necrosis and lead to abscess formation.
  - Managed with IV antibiotics and urgent surgical debridement.

- Pancreatic pseudocysts:
  - May be complicated by haemorrhage into a cyst, infection or rarely by rupture causing pancreatic ascites.
- Respiratory failure due to acute respiratory distress syndrome (ARDS).
- Disseminated intravascular coagulation.
- Shock/renal failure.
- Portal vein/splenic vein thrombosis leading to gastric varices.

PROGNOSIS

- Calculated using the Modified Glasgow Score (see MICRO-facts box):
  - Score of ≥3 is indicative of severe pancreatitis.

MICRO-facts

Glasgow scoring system

Three or more of the following factors within 48 hours of onset suggest severe pancreatitis and the need for prophylactic antibiotics and high dependency care:

PaO$_2$ <8 kPa
Age >55 years
Neutrophils: white cell count (WCC) >15 ×10^9/L
Calcium <2 mmol/L
Renal function: urea >16 mmol/L
Enzymes: lactate dehydrogenase (LDH) >600 IU/L, aspartate amino-transferase (AST) >200 IU/L
Albumin >32 g/L
Sugar: glucose >10 mmol/L

9.7 CHRONIC PANCREATITIS

DEFINITION

- Progressive inflammation of the pancreas that worsens over an extended period of time leading to irreversible damage.

AETIOLOGY

- Long-standing alcohol abuse (most common cause).
- Gallstones.
- Autoimmune pancreatitis:
  - Inflammation of the pancreas by lymphoplasmacytoid cells associated with raised gamma-globulins (Ig4). Can be associated with PSC.
- Haemochromatosis.
- Cystic fibrosis.

- Malignant obstruction:
  - Ampullary adenomas.
  - Carcinoma.
  - Pancreatic tumours.
- Idiopathic (may be due to genetic causes).

CLINICAL FEATURES

- History:
  - Chronic pain (intermittent or continuous).
  - Steatorrhoea: occurs when lipase levels fall to less than 10%.
  - Weight loss (due to malabsorption).
  - Symptoms of B_{12} deficiency (see Section 6.5).

INVESTIGATIONS

- As for acute pancreatitis (see Section 9.6):
  - Serum amylase and lipase may not be raised in chronic pancreatitis.
- Blood tests:
  - Serum IgG4:
    - Used to screen for autoimmune pancreatitis (elevated in up to 2/3 of patients).
    - May occasionally also be elevated in cases of pancreatic carcinoma.
  - Glucose levels.
  - Fat-soluble vitamin levels (vitamins A, D and E, and a prothrombin time).
  - Vitamin B_{12} level.
- Faecal elastase: low levels suggest pancreatic insufficiency.
- AXR: shows pancreatic calcification in 30% of advanced cases.
- CT scan.
- MRCP.
- EUS/biopsy (useful in differentiating pancreatic masses):
  - Will show histological features of chronic pancreatitis including inflammation, fibrosis and calcification of tissue.
  - Useful for confirming a diagnosis of autoimmune pancreatitis or excluding malignancy.

MANAGEMENT

- Lifestyle modification:
  - Avoidance of precipitants: alcohol, smoking etc.
- Pharmacological intervention:
  - Pain management:
    - Opioids often required.
    - Pancreatic enzyme supplements: suppress production of endogenous pancreatic enzymes, reducing ductal pressure.
    - Nerve blocks: coeliac axis/splanchnic nerve blocks.

- ERCP:
  - Temporary pancreatic duct stenting.
  - Removal of proximal pancreatic duct stones.
  - Pancreatic sphincterotomy.
- Surgical procedures:
  - Drainage of pancreatic duct.
  - Partial pancreatectomy/total pancreatectomy.
- Management of steatorrhoea:
  - Enzyme supplements with meals.
- Management of any underlying condition:
  - Corticosteroids/immunosuppression for autoimmune pancreatitis.

9.8 PANCREATIC CANCER

EPIDEMIOLOGY

- Pancreatic cancer is the fifth most common cause of death from cancer in the UK.
- Approximately 95% of pancreatic malignancies are adenocarcinomas.
- The 5-year survival rate following presentation is approximately 3%.

RISK FACTORS

- Older age: most patients present over the age of 60 years.
- Smoking.
- Diabetes mellitus.
- Obesity (high intake of fat/meat).
- Chronic pancreatitis.
- Hereditary pancreatitis (up to 40% develop pancreatic cancer by age 70).
- Peutz–Jeghers syndrome.

PATHOPHYSIOLOGY

- Arises from cells of the pancreatic duct in 85–90% of cases.
- Carcinoma may arise from any anatomical region of the pancreas: head, body or tail of the pancreas:
  - 60% occur in the head of the pancreas.
- Pancreatic carcinoma commonly spreads to:
  - Portal and mesenteric vessels (owing to their proximity).
  - Regional lymph nodes.
  - Liver.
- Due to the silent nature of the condition, metastases are often already present at diagnosis.

CLINICAL FEATURES

- History:
  - Painless jaundice: characteristic of carcinoma of the head of the pancreas.
  - Abdominal pain:
    - Epigastric pain radiating to the back.
    - Pain is more severe when the patient lies flat.
  - Anorexia/weight loss.
  - Steatorrhoea/features of malabsorption.
  - Recent onset of diabetes.
- Examination:
  - Palpable abdominal mass.
  - Hepatomegaly.
  - Palpable gallbladder:
    - In the presence of obstructive jaundice, this is known as Courvoisier's sign.
  - Thrombophlebitis migrans (Trousseau's sign):
    - Transient swelling and redness of different veins in the limbs due to the formation of clots associated with malignancy.

INVESTIGATIONS

- Blood tests:
  - FBC: normochromic anaemia.
  - LFTs: cholestatic pattern.
  - CA 19-9:
    - Tumour marker for pancreatic and hepatobiliary malignancies.
    - May be used to assess patient's response to ongoing treatment.
- Abdominal ultrasound scan: able to detect the majority of pancreatic carcinomas.
- CT scan: used for staging of pancreatic carcinoma (see MICRO-reference box).
- MRCP scan.
- EUS: allows for biopsy of lesions.

> **MICRO-reference**
> For further information on the staging of pancreatic cancer, see:
> http://www.cancer.org/cancer/pancreaticcancer/detailedguide/
> pancreatic-cancer-staging

Gastroenterology

MANAGEMENT

- Surgical intervention:
  - Pancreaticoduodenectomy (Whipple's procedure):
    - Removal of the head of the pancreas, gallbladder, duodenum and bile duct, usually with preservation of the pylorus/distal stomach.
    - Anastomosis is formed between the rest of the pancreas and jejunum, and the proximal bile duct and jejunum.
  - Palliative surgery:
    - Enteral stent insertion or bypass to relieve intestinal obstruction.
    - Biliary stent insertion to relieve jaundice (usually at ERCP).
- Pharmacological intervention:
  - Palliative chemotherapy (gemcitabine).

COMPLICATIONS

- Pancreatic insufficiency:
  - Pancreatic enzyme supplements and a high-calorie diet may help to reduce weight loss.
- Intestinal obstruction.
- Biliary obstruction.
- Severe abdominal pain:
  - May be difficult to control.
  - Opiates and radiotherapy may be considered to manage pain.

PROGNOSIS

- Pancreatic carcinoma carries an extremely poor prognosis:
  - Only 20% of patients will be suitable for surgery on presentation, with a 5-year survival rate of 10%.
  - The 5-year survival rate overall is approximately 5%.

MICRO-case

A 67-year-old publican presents to the ED with severe abdominal pain that becomes unbearable when he attempts to lie down for examination. His wife reports that he has vomited twice that morning. When questioned about his alcohol intake, the patient admits that he regularly drinks in the evenings, but denies that he has a problem.

The doctor prescribes morphine for pain relief before performing an abdominal examination, keeping the patient at an upward angle to prevent exacerbation of his abdominal pain. Examination reveals epigastric tenderness, but no signs of peritonism or jaundice. He has not had similar pains before. The junior doctor in the ED orders a number of blood

continued...

Gastroenterology

continued...

tests, including U&Es, which show a urea of 18 mmol/L, an FBC showing a WCC of 16×10^9/L and serum amylase level, which is 1230 U/mL.

Suspecting that the patient is suffering from acute pancreatitis, the doctor organizes further blood tests to assess the severity of the pancreatitis using the Modified Glasgow Score. The patient's oxygen saturations are normal, and further blood tests are ordered including LFTs, blood glucose and a lactate dehydrogenase (LDH) level. An abdominal ultrasound is also performed to look for underlying causes and exclude complications such as pseudocysts.

Later, the junior doctor receives the results of the patient's LFTs, and LDH, which show: bilirubin 22 μmol/L, ALT 78 IU/L, ALP 110 IU/L, γGT 450 IU/L, albumin 35 g/L and LDH 700 IU/L.

His Modified Glasgow Score is 4 and he is transferred to the high dependency unit for intensive monitoring.

Key points:

- Although gallstones are the most common underlying aetiology for acute pancreatitis, alcohol abuse is also a common cause.
- Diagnosis of acute pancreatitis is suggested by a serum amylase at least three times the normal range.
- When taking a medical history in cases of suspected pancreatitis, a history of the patient's alcoholic intake must be ascertained.
- All cases of acute pancreatitis should be graded by using a scoring system such as the Modified Glasgow Score.
- A disproportionally high γGT is suggestive of alcohol excess.
- An ultrasound is useful to look for gallstones, bile duct obstruction and complications such as pseudocysts.

10

Liver disease

10.1 ANATOMY

ANATOMY OF THE LIVER

- Lobes:
  - Anatomical:
    - The liver is split into the right and left lobes, which are separated by the falciform ligament.
    - The larger right lobe is further divided into the caudate and quadrate lobes.
  - Functional:
    - The liver can also be separated into two roughly equal functional lobes (right and left).
    - The division of these lobes occurs along the line running from the inferior vena cava (IVC) to the gallbladder.
    - The Couinaud classification of liver anatomy further subdivides the liver into eight segments, each containing:
      - A branch of the biliary tree.
      - A branch of the hepatic artery.
      - A branch of the hepatic portal vein.
- Lobules:
  - The lobes of the liver are further subdivided into lobules.
  - These are composed of a number of acini:
    - Functional units of the liver comprised a central vein surrounded by hepatocytes.
- Ligaments:
  - Falciform ligament:
    - Embryological remnant of the umbilical vein.
    - Forms an attachment between the anterior abdominal wall and the liver.
    - Becomes continuous with the coronary ligament at the diaphragm.

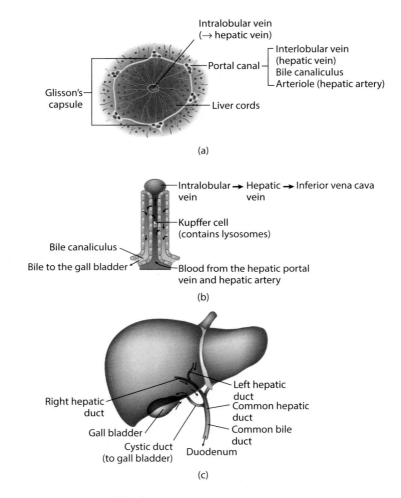

Figure 10.1 **Anatomy of the liver.**

- Ligamentum teres (round ligament):
  - Divides the left lobe of the liver into medial and lateral sections.
  - Embryological remnant of the umbilical vein.
- Coronary ligament:
  - Forms an attachment between the diaphragm and the superior aspect of the liver.
  - Along with the IVC, forms the boundary of the 'bare area' of the liver (the only area of the liver not covered by peritoneum).
- Ligamentum venosum:
  - Embryological remnant of the ductus venosus.

- Vasculature:
  - Blood supply to the liver is from two main sources:
    - Hepatic artery (30% of blood supply):
      - Provides oxygenated blood to the liver.
    - Hepatic portal vein (70% of blood supply):
      - Provides deoxygenated, nutrient-rich blood from the GI tract.
      - Drains to the hepatic veins, which drain to the IVC.
  - Blood vessels enter the liver at the porta hepatis, which contains:
    - Hepatic portal vein.
    - Hepatic arteries (right and left).
    - Common bile duct.

FUNCTIONS OF THE LIVER

- Metabolism:
  - Carbohydrates:
    - The liver can convert excess glucose into glycogen (glycogenesis) for storage or fatty acids for storage in adipose tissue.
    - Glycogen stores can be broken down to glucose (glycogenolysis) when blood glucose levels are low.
    - When glycogen stores are depleted, the liver can synthesize glucose from amino acids and lactate (gluconeogenesis).
  - Protein:
    - Deamination of excess amino acids, producing ammonia as a by-product.
    - Conversion of ammonia to urea via the ornithine cycle.
    - The kidneys excrete the urea.
  - Lipids:
    - Synthesis of bile acids to aid the formation of micelles for lipid absorption.
    - Cholesterol and lipoprotein synthesis.
    - Processes chylomicrons with subsequent formation of VLDL.
    - Oxidation of triglycerides to produce energy.
  - Bilirubin:
    - Conjugation of bilirubin and excretion via the biliary system.
- Synthesis:
  - Production of coagulation factors: I, II, V, VII, IX, X and XI.
  - Production of plasma proteins: e.g. albumin.
- Storage:
  - Glycogen.
  - Vitamins: A, D, B_{12}.
  - Iron.
- Detoxification:
  - Drug and alcohol metabolism.
  - Hormone metabolism (e.g. insulin, glucocorticoids).

Gastroenterology

10.2 VIRAL HEPATITIS

DEFINITION

- Inflammation of the liver due to infection with hepatotropic viruses (e.g. hepatitis A, B, C, D, E).
- Viral hepatitis can also result from systemic infection with CMV, EBV or herpes simplex.

HEPATITIS A

- A 28-nm non-enveloped RNA virus of the picornavirus family.
- Transmission is via faecal–oral route:
  - 1.5 million symptomatic cases per year, generally occurring in areas of poor sanitation in association with contaminated water.
- Incubation period of approximately 2–4 weeks.
- Clinical features:
  - History:
    - Fatigue.
    - Fever: generally low grade.
    - Nausea and vomiting.
    - Anorexia.
    - Abdominal pain.
    - Myalgia.
  - Examination:
    - Hepatomegaly.
    - Jaundice.
    - Pale stools/dark urine.
- Investigations:
  - Blood tests:
    - FBC: lymphocytosis.
    - LFTs: ↑ AST/ALT.
  - Serology:
    - IgM anti-HAV antibodies are present at diagnosis and persist for 4 months.
    - IgG: anti-HAV antibodies often remain for life, signify past infection.
- Management:
  - Complete abstinence from alcohol.
  - Supportive treatment:
    - IV fluids.
    - Antiemetic medication.
    - Analgesia.
- Prevention:
  - Vaccination given to at-risk groups (travellers etc.).

- Prognosis:
  - Generally self-limiting.
  - Does not cause chronic infection.
  - Rarely causes fulminant hepatitis.
  - Patients may suffer a relapse of hepatitis A (rare).

HEPATITIS B

- A 42-nm enveloped DNA virus of the Hepadnaviridae family.
- Approximately 400 million people are infected worldwide.
- Endemic in Southeast Asia and sub-Saharan Africa.
- Transmission is via:
  - Blood-borne spread:
    - Contaminated blood products.
    - IV drug use.
  - Sexual contact:
    - Increased risk in men who have sex with men.
  - Vertical transmission (from mother to neonate during delivery):
    - Most common route.
  - Breast milk.
- Incubation period of approximately 2–3 months.
- Clinical features:
  - History:
    - Fever.
    - Nausea and vomiting.
    - Abdominal pain: right upper quadrant.
    - Anorexia.
    - Arthralgia.
  - Examination:
    - Rash (generally urticarial).
    - Jaundice (30% of cases).
    - Dark urine.
    - Pale stools.
    - Signs of chronic liver disease (in patients with chronic infection).
- Investigations:
  - Blood tests:
    - LFTs: ↑ ALT/AST.
  - Serology (also see MICRO-facts box):
    - Hepatitis B surface antigen (HBsAg):
      - Surface protein of the hepatitis B virus.
      - Detected approximately 6–8 weeks after exposure.
      - Indicates patient is suffering from chronic hepatitis B if present >6 months after initial infection.

Gastroenterology

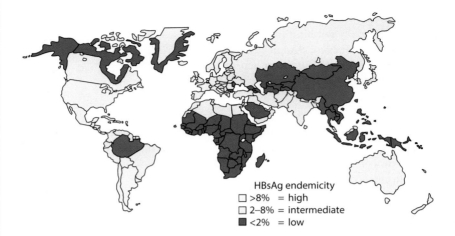

Figure 10.2 Map of the world showing areas endemic for hepatitis B.

- – Hepatitis B envelope antigen (HBeAg):
  - ○ Indicates high rate of viral replication and infectivity.
- – Hepatitis B core antibody (HBcAb) suggests latent infection.
- – Hepatitis B surface antibody (anti-HBs):
  - ○ Immunological response to the presence of HBsAg.
  - ○ Indicates recovery in a patient with hepatitis B.
  - ○ Also present in patients who have been vaccinated against hepatitis B.
- Imaging (indicated in patients with chronic disease):
  - – Fibroscan: non-invasive measure of fibrosis.
  - – Ultrasound scan (USS).
  - – CT scan.
  - – MRI.
- Liver biopsy: to assess degree of inflammation and fibrosis.

MICRO-facts

The following table shows the serological profiles of different patients with different exposures to hepatitis B virus.

ANTIBODY/ANTIGEN	PATIENT				
	1	2	3	4	5
Anti-HBc IgM	–ve	+ve	–ve	–ve	–ve
Anti-HBc IgG	–ve	–ve	+ve	+ve	+ve

continued...

continued...

ANTIBODY/ANTIGEN	PATIENT				
	1	2	3	4	5
HBeAg	−ve	+ve	+ve	−ve	−ve
HBeAb	−ve	−ve	+ve	+ve	+ve
HBsAg	−ve	+ve	+ve	+ve	−ve
HBsAb	+ve	−ve	−ve	−ve	+ve
Hep B Viral Load	−ve	High	High	Low	−ve
ALT	Normal	Raised	Raised	Fluctuating	Normal

Patient 1:

This patient is a surface antibody carrier, meaning that the patient has been previously immunized against the infection.

Patient 2:

This patient is suffering from an acute infection of hepatitis B, illustrated by the presence of the IgM antibody against the core antigen. In the later stages of infection, HBc IgG antibodies appear as the IgM antibodies disappear, approximately 6 months after the onset of infection. HBe antigen signifies high viral replication and high infectivity.

Patient 3:

This patient has chronic hepatitis B, characterized by the persistence of HBsAg for more than 6 months. The patient has high viral titres suggested by the presence of HBe antigen, and will suffer ongoing liver damage without treatment.

Patient 4:

This patient also has chronic hepatitis B. The patient has low viral levels as suggested by loss of the HBe antigen and development of the HBe antibody. This usually represents a later stage of infection and such patients often have mildly fluctuating LFTs. In these cases, liver injury occurs very slowly if at all.

Patient 5:

This patient has cleared the hepatitis B infection and developed immunity against the infection as seen by the development of HBs antibodies. HBe antibodies usually disappear from the blood over time.

- Management:
  - Complete abstinence from alcohol.
  - Supportive treatment.
  - Contact tracing.

Gastroenterology

- Chronic hepatitis:
  - Pegylated interferon-α (often poorly tolerated):
    - Administered by weekly injection for 48 weeks.
    - Leads to a significant suppression of hepatitis B in 25–60%.
  - Nucleoside analogues: e.g. tenofovir, lamivudine:
    - Well-tolerated oral agents usually taken long-term.
    - Tenofovir causes significant viral suppression in 74–90%.
- Prevention:
  - Vaccination given to at-risk groups (healthcare professionals etc.).
- Complications:
  - Chronic hepatitis B:
    - Occurs in approximately 5–10% of patients.
  - Cirrhosis.
  - Glomerulonephritis.
  - Polyarteritis nodosa.
  - Fulminant liver failure.
  - Infection with hepatitis D virus.
  - Increased risk of heptatocellular carcinoma.
- Prognosis:
  - 90–95% of cases resolve spontaneously.
  - 5–10% develop chronic hepatitis of whom 10–20% will develop cirrhosis within 5 years of diagnosis.

HEPATITIS C

- A 55-nm, enveloped, single-stranded RNA virus of the Flavivirus family.
- Approximately 170 million cases worldwide.
- High incidence in North Africa.
- Transmission: as for hepatitis B.
- Incubation period of 6–8 weeks.
- Clinical features:
  - Mostly asymptomatic.
  - History:
    - Malaise.
    - Pruritis.
    - Arthralgia/myalgia.
    - Abdominal pain.
  - Examination:
    - Jaundice occurs in 10–20% of acute cases.
    - Signs of chronic liver disease (see Section 4.2).
- Investigations:
  - LFTs.

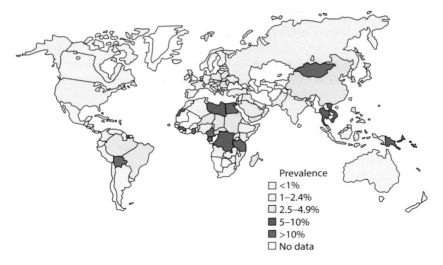

Figure 10.3 Map of the world showing areas endemic for hepatitis C.

- Serology:
  - Hepatitis C antibody: becomes positive approximately 2 weeks after the onset of symptoms.
  - PCR for the detection of hepatitis C viral RNA.
  - Genotype testing (determines treatment).
- Imaging:
  - USS (used to demonstrate cirrhosis in chronic hepatitis).
  - Fibroscan (detection of cirrhosis/fibrosis).
- Liver biopsy:
  - Used to discover the extent of the damage to the liver.
- Management:
  - Pegylated interferon-α.
  - Ribavirin.
  - Protease inhibitors (telaprevir, boceprevir, simeprevir) for genotype 1.
  - Recently developed oral direct-acting antivirals:
    - Allow treatment of hepatitis C without the use of pegylated interferon.
    - Clearance rates of up to 95%.
- Prevention:
  - Avoidance of risk factors.
  - There is currently no vaccination available for hepatitis C.
- Complications:
  - Cirrhosis: 10–40% of patients develop cirrhosis after 20–30 years.
  - Glomerulonephritis.

Gastroenterology

- Essential cryoglobulinaemia.
- Increased risk of hepatocellular carcinoma (HCC).
- Prognosis:
  - Much higher incidence of chronic hepatitis than with hepatitis B (80%).
  - The virus can be eradicated with treatment in around 70% of patients.

HEPATITIS D

- A 1.7-kb, single-stranded RNA satellite virus that utilizes HBsAg in its envelope.
- Transmission:
  - Contracted by individuals who are already infected with hepatitis B virus.
- Incubation period of approximately 4–5 weeks.
- Clinical features:
  - When contracted alongside an acute hepatitis B infection, causes a more severe form of acute hepatitis.
  - When contracted in a chronic carrier of hepatitis B, causes an acute-on-chronic presentation of hepatitis.
- Investigations:
  - Serology:
    - Hepatitis D antibody.
- Management:
  - Pegylated interferon-α.

HEPATITIS E

- A 32-nm RNA virus of the hepatitis E like viral family.
- Transmission is via the faecal–oral route.
- Endemic in areas with poor sanitation (e.g. Southeast Asia, Northern and Central Africa, Central America and the Middle East).
- Incubation period of 2–10 weeks.
- Clinical features:
  - Mostly asymptomatic in children.
  - Similar presentation to that of hepatitis A.
  - High mortality rates among pregnant women (15–25%).
- Investigations:
  - Serology:
    - Hepatitis E IgM, IgG antibody.
- Management:
  - Supportive treatment.
- Prevention:
  - Good standards of hygiene and sanitation.

10.3 AUTOIMMUNE HEPATITIS

DEFINITION

- Inflammation of the liver associated with hypergammaglobulinaemia, autoantibodies and interface hepatitis on histology.
- Type 1 autoimmune hepatitis:
  - Most common form.
  - Associated with antinuclear antibodies and/or smooth muscle antibodies.
- Type 2 autoimmune hepatitis:
  - More common in young female patients.
  - Greater association with history of other autoimmune conditions.
  - Associated with anti-LKM antibodies.

RISK FACTORS

- Prevalence of 10–15 cases per 100,000.
- Female gender (3:1).
- Past medical history of other autoimmune conditions: e.g. autoimmune thyroiditis.
- HLA associations (B8, DR3, DR4).
- Medications: e.g. statins, hydralazine, nitrofurantoin, minocycline.

CLINICAL FEATURES

- History: clinical features of acute hepatitis (see above):
  - 30% asymptomatic (diagnosed on blood testing).
  - 20% present with decompensated liver disease.
- Examination:
  - Jaundice.
  - Hepatomegaly ± splenomegaly.
- Associated conditions:
  - Autoimmune thyroiditis.
  - Membranoproliferative glomerulonephritis.
  - Ulcerative colitis.
  - Rheumatoid arthritis.
  - Coeliac disease.

INVESTIGATIONS

- Blood tests:
  - LFTs: ↑ AST/ALT, ↑ IgG.
  - Autoantibodies:
    - Antinuclear antibody (ANA).
    - Anti-smooth muscle antibody.

Gastroenterology

- Soluble liver antigens: e.g. anti-asialoglycoprotein receptor antibody.
- Anti- LKM1: associated with type 2 autoimmune hepatitis.
- USS: to look for evidence of cirrhosis/complications of cirrhosis.
- Liver biopsy:
  - Infiltration with lymphocytes and plasma cells causing interface hepatitis.
  - Fibrosis and necrosis in advanced disease.

MANAGEMENT

- Induction of remission:
  - Prednisolone/budesonide used to induce remission.
  - Azathioprine added as a steroid sparing agent.
  - In those who fail to respond, high-dose azathioprine, mycophenolate or tacrolimus has been used.
- Liver transplant:
  - Used in patients who do not respond to medical management.

PROGNOSIS

- Majority of patients achieve remission with immunosuppressive medication.
- In those who achieve remission, 50–90% will relapse on stopping therapy within 12 months.

10.4 PRIMARY BILIARY CIRRHOSIS

DEFINITION

- Gradual destruction of the intralobular bile ducts resulting in chronic cholestasis commonly associated with anti-mitochondrial antibodies.

EPIDEMIOLOGY

- Prevalence of approximately 6–10 in 100,000.

RISK FACTORS

- Female gender (10 females affected to 1 male).
- Age >40 years.
- Other autoimmune conditions (autoimmune thyroiditis, renal tubular acidosis, Sjögren's syndrome etc.).

CLINICAL FEATURES

- May be asymptomatic.
- History:
  - Fatigue.
  - Pruritis.
  - Abdominal pain (right upper quadrant).

- Examination:
  - Jaundice.
  - Hepatomegaly ± splenomegaly.
  - Skin pigmentation (due to increased melanin).
  - Cholesterol deposits: xanthelasma etc.
  - Pale stools/dark urine.

INVESTIGATIONS

- Blood tests:
  - LFTs: ↑ ALP, ↑ γGT.
  - ↑ IgM.
  - Autoantibodies:
    - Anti-mitochondrial antibodies (95%).
  - Serum cholesterol: increased (no increase in cardiovascular disease).
- Imaging:
  - Used to exclude differential diagnoses and for detection of cirrhosis.
- Liver biopsy:
  - Periportal lymphocyte infiltration and destruction of the bile ducts with non-caseating granulomas progressing to fibrosis and cirrhosis.

MANAGEMENT

- Pharmacological intervention:
  - Ursodeoxycholic acid.
  - Management of pruritis:
    - Bile salt sequestrants (e.g. cholestyramine/colesevelam)
    - Rifampicin.
    - Naltrexone.
  - Supplementation of fat-soluble vitamins (A, D, E and K).
- Liver transplant: indicated in end-stage disease.

COMPLICATIONS

- Osteoporosis: bisphosphonates often used in these patients.
- Portal hypertension.
- Decompensated liver disease/HCC.

10.5 PRIMARY SCLEROSING CHOLANGITIS

DEFINITION

- Inflammation and progressive fibrosis of the intra- and extrahepatic bile ducts leading to their destruction and chronic cholestasis.

Gastroenterology

EPIDEMIOLOGY

- Rare condition: prevalence of approximately 8/100,000.
- More common in men (2:1).
- Typical presentation is at 40 years.
- Approximately 80% of cases have concomitant IBD and HIV.
- Genetic component: association with certain HLA types: DR3, A1, B8.

CLINICAL FEATURES

- May be asymptomatic (discovered on incidental investigation)
- History:
    - Abdominal pain (right upper quadrant)
    - Pruritis.
    - Weight loss.
    - Fatigue.
    - Fever.
- Examination:
    - Jaundice.
    - Hepatomegaly ± splenomegaly.
    - Signs of liver disease (in advanced cases).

INVESTIGATIONS

- Blood tests:
    - LFTs:
        - ↑ ALP, ↑ γGT, ↑ bilirubin.
    - Autoantibodies:
        - Perinuclear antineutrophil cytoplasmic antibodies.
        - Other autoantibodies may be present but are not diagnostic (e.g. ANA).
- Imaging:
    - Abdominal USS.
    - MRCP.
    - ERCP: brushings of dominant stricture to exclude cholangiocarcinoma.
- Biopsy:
    - Fibro-obliteration of medium-sized bile ducts with fibrosis spreading into the liver lobules in more advanced disease.

MANAGEMENT

- Pharmacological intervention:
    - Ursodeoxycholic acid.
    - Treatment of pruritis (see Section 10.4).

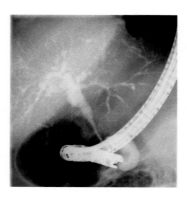

Figure 10.4 Endoscopic retrograde cholangiopancreatography (ERCP) showing primary sclerosing cholangitis.

- Antibiotics:
  - Given if clinical suspicion of bacterial cholangitis (e.g. co-amoxiclav, ciprofloxacin).
- Surgical intervention:
  - Endoscopic dilatation and stenting of biliary strictures.
  - Surgical resection of strictures/liver transplantation.

COMPLICATIONS

- Bacterial cholangitis:
  - May occur following formation of a biliary stricture or after endoscopic intervention.
- Increased incidence of gallstones (often pigment stones).
- Portal hypertension.
- Cirrhosis.
- Increased risk of cholangiocarcinoma.
- Metabolic bone disease.
- Ulcerative colitis/colorectal cancer (patients with IBD/PSC require annual colonoscopy).

10.6 DRUG-INDUCED LIVER INJURY

DEFINITION

- Liver damage and/or dysfunction secondary to exposure to a causative drug.

EPIDEMIOLOGY

- Drug-induced liver injury is the major cause of acute liver failure:
  - Most commonly secondary to paracetamol overdose.

Gastroenterology

PATHOLOGY

- The liver is a major site of drug detoxification, metabolism and elimination.
- Damage occurs due to a range of different processes including:
  - Direct toxicity.
  - Autoimmune reaction to hepatocytes expressing drug metabolites.
  - Disruption of cellular calcium homeostasis.
  - Generation of free radicals.
  - Metabolism of drug to toxic metabolites.
- Effects can be dose dependent or idiosyncratic (non-dose dependent):
  - Dose dependent: effects are related to the dose of the drug and are therefore predictable.
  - Idiosyncratic: effects can happen at any dose and are difficult to predict:
    - May be a latent period between drug administration and liver damage.
- See Table 10.1 for details of common causative drugs and their effects.

CLINICAL FEATURES

- Signs and symptoms are a result of the underlying damage and can therefore vary between drugs.

Table 10.1 **Drug-induced liver injury: pathological changes and causative agents**

PATHOLOGY	DRUG
Hepatitis (acute or chronic)	Isoniazid, indomethacin, phenytoin, nitrofurantoin, rifampicin, methyldopa, atenolol, verapamil/enalapril, volatile inhalational anaesthetic agents (halothane), methyldopa
Steatohepatitis	Amiodarone, nifedipine
Cholestasis	Oral contraceptive pill, haloperidol, chlorpromazine, erythromycin, anabolic steroids, allopurinol, co-amoxiclav, carbamazepine, azathioprine, flucloxacillin, oral hypoglycaemics
Fibrosis	Methotrexate, alcohol, isoniazid, vitamin A, arsenic, α-methyldopa
Zone necrosis	Paracetamol, cocaine, carbon tetrachloride, salicylates
Oncogenic	Oral contraceptive pill, oestrogens, danazol, anabolic steroids

Gastroenterology

- Any patient with liver symptoms should have a detailed drug history taken including:
  - Current medications including non-prescribed medications.
  - Recent dose changes/new drugs – dose-dependent reaction.
  - Any other drugs taken in last few months – idiosyncratic reaction.

MANAGEMENT

- Specific management depending on the drug (e.g. *N*-acetylcysteine for paracetamol).
- In all cases, once identified, the causative drug should be stopped.
- Supportive treatment may be required.
- Further drug prescribing should take into account the patients previous reaction.

MICRO-facts

Paracetamol shows a dose-dependent reaction and can progress to acute liver failure very quickly. Blood paracetamol levels should be taken from patients with suspected or known overdoses 4 hours post ingestion. The paracetamol level is then plotted on a chart (nomogram) to influence management. A treatment line on the chart shows which patients need treatment and which patients are at low risk of liver failure and therefore need no treatment.

10.7 ALCOHOL-RELATED LIVER DISEASE

DEFINITION

- Damage to the liver caused by long-term heavy alcohol (ethanol) consumption.
- There are a range of manifestations:
  - Steatosis – fatty changes in the liver.
  - Steatohepatitis – fatty changes and inflammation.
  - Cirrhosis – scarring (fibrosis) of the liver.

EPIDEMIOLOGY

- Steatosis can be found in 90% of heavy drinkers: reverses with abstinence.
- Up to a third of heavy drinkers will progress to steatohepatits.
- Cirrhosis occurs in less than 20% of heavy drinkers: can regress with abstinence.

> **MICRO-reference**
> A report in 2009 estimated that 24% of the population in England drinks to a potentially harmful level (33% of men, 16% of women), while 6% demonstrates alcohol dependence (9% men, 3% women). See: http://www.esds.ac.uk/doc/6379/mrdoc/pdf/6379research_report.pdf

RISK FACTORS

- Duration of alcohol abuse: >20 years is high risk.
- Female gender.
- Obesity: increases risk of liver disease two- to threefold.
- Smoking.
- Genetic factors:
  - Genetic polymorphisms in alcohol metabolism (CYP2E1).
- Comorbid hepatitis C infection (see Section 10.2) or haemochromatosis (see Section 10.9).

PATHOPHYSIOLOGY

- Alcohol causes fat to accumulate in the liver (steatosis) in two ways:
  - Oxidation of alcohol causes disruption of carbohydrate metabolism and increases fatty acid production.
  - Energy which would have been used to oxidize fatty acids is diverted into alcohol metabolism, leading to decreased metabolism of fatty acids.
- Steatohepatitis may be caused by several mechanisms:
  - Acetaldehyde production:
    - Acetaldehyde is a by-product of alcohol metabolism.
    - Binds to hepatocyte proteins affecting their biological function.
  - Oxidative stress:
    - Caused by alcohol.
  - Mitochondrial dysfunction:
    - Impaired glutathione transport increases damage from oxidative stress.
  - Hypoxia:
    - Caused by increased oxygen demand in alcohol metabolism.
- The long-term result of this liver damage is cirrhosis:
  - Damaged hepatocytes try to regenerate but the structure of the liver is lost.

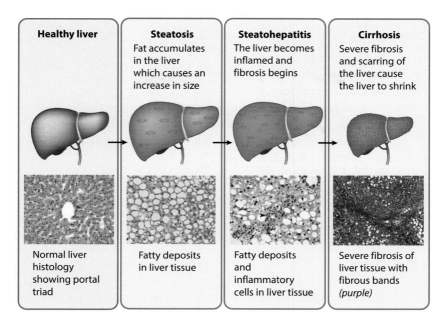

Figure 10.5 Sequence of fatty changes in the liver.

- Collagen production causes fibrosis:
  - Cytokines produced as a result of oxidative stress cause hepatic stellate cells to become collagen-producing cells.
- Fibrous bands become incorporated into the architecture, separating the liver into nodules and disrupting blood supply.
- All of the changes listed above can disrupt the normal function of the liver to varying degrees.

CLINICAL FEATURES

- History:
  - Steatosis is usually asymptomatic.
  - Steatohepatitis can be asymptomatic or may present with features of alcoholic hepatitis (general malaise, jaundice, ascites).
  - Cirrhosis is initially usually asymptomatic:
    - Superimposed steatohepatitis or advanced cirrhosis can result in decompensation.
- Examination:
  - Hepatomegaly is common ± splenomegaly.

Gastroenterology

- Jaundice.
- Ascites.
- Ankle oedema.
- Stigmata of chronic liver disease:
  - Palmar erythema.
  - Spider naevi: dilated arteriole with characteristic red radiations.
  - Gynaecomastia: breast tissue enlargement in males.
  - Caput medusa: distension of abdominal veins around umbilicus.
- Associated features of alcohol abuse:
  - Signs of dependency (see Section 4.3).
  - Poor nutritional status.
  - Poor self-care.

INVESTIGATIONS

- Blood tests:
  - LFTs:
    - AST and ALT are raised in steatohepatitis (usually AST > ALT).
    - γGT is sensitive but not specific for alcohol use.
    - In severe disease, ALP, prothrombin time (PT) and serum bilirubin are all raised.
    - Albumin may be low.
  - FBC: raised MCV.
- Imaging:
  - USS of the liver shows fatty infiltration (bright, echogenic appearance).
  - May also show fibrosis and scarring if patient has progressed to cirrhosis.
- Fibroscan: non-invasive assessment of fibrosis.
- Ascitic tap if the patient has ascites:
  - Send for microscopy (differential white cell count and gram stain), culture and sensitivities (MC+S), as there is an increased risk of spontaneous bacterial peritonitis (SBP).
- Liver biopsy:
  - Histology can confirm diagnosis:
    - Balloon degeneration of hepatocytes.
    - Mallory's hyaline.
    - Megamitochondria.
    - Centrilobular, macrovesicular fatty infiltration.
    - Fibrosis may also be present.

MANAGEMENT

- Lifestyle modifications:
  - Cessation of alcohol consumption: risk of delirium tremens.
- Pharmacological intervention:
  - Treatment of nutritional deficiencies: vitamin supplementation with thiamine, folate, B vitamins.
  - Management of ascites (see complications below): diuretics/paracentesis.
  - Treatment of severe alcoholic hepatitis: Maddrey's score ≥32 (see below):
    - Corticosteroids.
    - Pentoxyfyline (anti-TNF).
  - Maintaining alcohol abstinence:
    - Disulfiram: reacts with alcohol causing an accumulation of acetaldehyde causing flushing, nausea, vomiting, palpitations and dizziness.
    - Acamprosate: reduces craving for alcohol.
- Surgical intervention:
  - Liver transplantation: indicated in chronic disease:
    - Patients usually required to be abstinent from alcohol for at least 6 months.

MICRO-facts

Rapid cessation of alcohol consumption can result in delirium tremens. This is a potentially fatal condition characterized by confusion, agitation, tremors, hallucinations and possibly seizures. It is important to recognize and treat early (see Section 4.3).

COMPLICATIONS

- Hyponatraemia/renal dysfunction can occur from the ingestion of large amounts of dilute alcoholic drinks in patients with poor nutrition:
  - Symptoms of hyponatraemia include:
    - Dizziness.
    - Weakness.
    - Neurological impairment.
    - Seizures.
- Portal hypertension can occur secondary to reduced blood flow through the liver:
  - Backpressure occurs in the portal vasculature.
  - Can result in splenomegaly, oesophageal varices, anorectal varices, gastric varices and caput medusa.
  - Varices can rupture causing massive haemorrhage.

Gastroenterology

- Ascites can also result from portal hypertension and renal dysfunction:
  - Fluid builds up in the peritoneum.
  - Increases the risk of SBP and portal vein/splenic vein thromboses.
- HCC:
  - Heavy alcohol consumption is a major risk factor for HCC.
- Encephalopathy (see Section 4.2).

PROGNOSIS

- Alcoholic hepatitis:
  - Severe disease characterized by a range of findings from abnormal LFTs to jaundice and liver failure.
  - Severity calculated using Maddrey's discriminate function (DF):
    - DF = (4.6 × prothrombin time − control [seconds]) + serum bilirubin (mg/dL).
    - A value of >32 equates to severe disease.
  - Mild disease prognosis: 1-month mortality of 0–10%.
  - Severe disease prognosis: 1-month mortality of 35–45%.
- 5-year survival:
  - Fatty liver: 70–80%.
  - Alcoholic hepatitis or cirrhosis: 50–75%.
  - Cirrhosis combined with alcoholic hepatitis: 30–50%.

10.8 NON-ALCOHOLIC FATTY LIVER DISEASE

DEFINITION

- Steatosis, steatohepatitis and/or cirrhosis that is not caused by excessive alcohol consumption:
  - The histological changes are identical to alcoholic liver disease, the only discriminating factor being alcohol consumption.
- Terminology:
  - NAFLD – non-alcoholic fatty liver disease:
    - General term covering all changes as listed above.
  - NASH – non-alcoholic steatohepatitis:
    - Specific term meaning inflammation and fatty infiltration.

EPIDEMIOLOGY

- Estimated prevalence of 25% within the population:
  - Only a small proportion of these patients will develop NASH.
  - Fewer still will progress to cirrhosis.
- NAFLD is much more common in obese patients.

AETIOLOGY/RISK FACTORS

- Metabolic syndrome:
  - Impaired glucose tolerance/diabetes mellitus.
  - Central obesity.
  - Hypertension.
  - Dyslipidaemia.
- Rapid weight loss:
  - Secondary to high levels of free fatty acids from adipose tissue breakdown.
- Drugs: amiodarone, valproate, methotrexate, tamoxifen etc.
- Total parenteral nutrition.
- Polycystic ovary syndrome.

PATHOPHYSIOLOGY

- The pathological changes are identical to those of alcoholic liver disease (see Section 10.7).
- Excess fatty acids entering the liver saturate the liver's capacity:
  - Mitochondria are unable to metabolize them, resulting in steatosis.
- Insulin resistance may potentiate this effect:
  - Down-regulates mitochondrial fatty acid oxidation.
- Steatosis results in several cellular adaptations and altered signalling pathways:
  - These leave the hepatocytes vulnerable to a second hit mediated by oxidative stress, cytokine alteration etc.
  - The second hit can cause hepatocyte necrosis, inflammation and activation of the fibrogenic cascade.

CLINICAL FEATURES

- As for alcoholic liver disease except:
  - Low alcohol consumption.
  - May be a history of diabetes.
- Examination:
  - Obesity.
  - Hypertension.

INVESTIGATIONS

- LFT:
  - As for alcoholic liver disease.
  - ALT often elevated more than AST.
  - γGT may be lower than in alcohol-related liver disease (ALD).

- Autoantibodies:
  - Up to 25% have a low titre of ANA.
- Glucose and lipids:
  - Both often elevated.
  - Diabetes or impaired glucose tolerance affects 20–75%.
- Ferritin:
  - Elevated in up to 50% of cases.
- Imaging:
  - USS: as for alcoholic liver disease.
  - CT/MRI for complications: e.g. liver lesions.
- Fibroscan: non-invasive assessment of fibrosis.
- Liver biopsy: confirmation of diagnosis.

MANAGEMENT

- Lifestyle modifications and management of risk factors:
  - Weight loss (aim for 1–2 lbs per week):
    - Low-fat, high-protein diet.
    - Exercise.
    - Orlistat – lipase inhibitor.
    - Bariatric surgery in complicated, difficult to manage cases.
  - Management of hypertension.
  - Diabetes mellitus/impaired glucose tolerance management:
    - Weight loss may be enough.
    - Metformin.
  - Hyperlipidaemia management – statins.
- Pharmacological interventions:
  - Insulin-sensitizing agents:
    - Metformin (although limited evidence).
    - Thiazolidinediones (e.g. rosiglitazone) – some benefit although associated with weight gain.
- Surgical intervention:
  - Transplantation:
    - Suitability depends on comorbidities such as vascular disease.

COMPLICATIONS

- Cirrhosis: increased risk if inflammation is present.
- Increased risk of HCC.

10.9 HEREDITARY HAEMOCHROMATOSIS

DEFINITION

- An inherited defect in iron metabolism leading to accumulation of iron in a range of tissues:
  - Liver.
  - Heart.
  - Pancreas.
  - Skin.
  - Brain.
  - Endocrine organs: e.g. gonads, thyroid and pituitary.

EPIDEMIOLOGY

- Most common in Northern Europe.
- More common in individuals of Irish/Celtic descent.

RISK FACTORS

- Co-existing causes of iron overload:
  - Iron-loading anaemia: thalassaemia, sideroblastic anaemia, chronic haemolytic anaemia etc.
  - Parenteral iron overload: multiple transfusions, iron infusions.
  - Chronic liver disease: hepatitis B and C, ALD.
  - Porphyria cutanea tarda.

PATHOPHYSIOLOGY

- Most commonly caused by a mutation of the HFE gene:
  - Shows autosomal recessive inheritance.
  - Heterozygotes have slightly dysfunctional iron metabolism but this does not lead to significant iron overload.
  - Homozygotes have increased iron absorption and deposition, which may lead to iron overload.
- A second mutation (H63D) can result in lesser degrees of increased iron absorption:
  - May result in iron overload if present in a heterozygotic individual.
- Iron metabolism is a complex and finely balanced process:
  - Ferric iron is reduced to ferrous and taken up by duodenal enterocytes and transported across the basolateral membrane to the plasma.
  - This process is regulated by a hepatic protein hepcidin which down-regulates absorption.
  - Mutation of the HFE gene results in low hepcidin levels and hence increased iron absorption.

Gastroenterology

- The mutant HFE gene increases intestinal iron absorption:
  - The iron transport protein (transferrin) is overloaded.
  - Free iron in the blood increases.
  - This excess iron is deposited over many years in several tissues including liver, pancreas and heart.
- Male homozygotes are at higher risk of iron overload than female homozygotes:
  - Menstruation is protective by removing iron from the body.

CLINICAL FEATURES

- History:
  - Non-specific symptoms of fatigue, weakness.
  - Symptoms of pituitary dysfunction: erectile dysfunction, infertility, amenorrhoea.
  - Symptoms of diabetes mellitus: polydipsia, polyuria, polyphagia.
  - Cardiac symptoms: heart failure, arrhythmias.
  - Joint pain due to chondrocalcinosis: commonly affects the knees and metacarpophalangeal joints.
  - Neurological symptoms: memory loss, depression.
- Examination:
  - Classic triad (only present in late disease):
    - Bronze skin.
    - Hepatomegaly.
    - Diabetes mellitus.
  - Arrhythmias.
  - Ankle/pulmonary oedema secondary to heart failure.

INVESTIGATIONS

- Iron studies:
  - Raised serum iron.
  - Reduced total iron-binding capacity (TIBC).
  - Raised ferritin.
- LFTs:
  - Often normal.
- Genetic analysis:
  - Screen patients with suspicious iron studies or those with unexplained chronic liver disease/family history.
- Liver biopsy:
  - Used to define the extent of tissue damage in the liver.
  - Not usually required for diagnosis.
- Endocrine investigations:
  - To assess damage to endocrine organs.

- Possible tests include blood glucose, oestrogen, testosterone, luteinising hormone, follicle-stimulating hormone, thyroid-stimulating hormone.

MANAGEMENT

- Venesection is the mainstay of management:
  - Initially, 500 mL of blood (around 250 mg iron) is removed every week/2 weeks.
  - Once serum iron, ferritin and MCV have normalized (aim for ferritin of 50–100 µg/L), venesection should be performed 3–4 times per year.
- Management of endocrine and cardiac complications.
- Liver transplant in patients with end-stage liver failure.
- Family screening:
  - Screen spouse of homozygote for C282Y mutation:
    - If they are a heterozygote, then children have a 50% chance of homozygosity.
  - Screen children:
    - Regular iron studies (annually) or genetic testing.
    - Genetic testing may be more cost effective.

COMPLICATIONS

- Increased risk of HCC.

10.10 WILSON'S DISEASE

DEFINITION

- An inherited defect of copper metabolism causing copper to accumulate in certain tissues.
- Also known as hepatolenticular degeneration.

PATHOPHYSIOLOGY

- Copper absorbed in the upper intestine is transported to the liver and other tissues bound to albumin:
  - Within the liver, copper is incorporated into apocaeruloplasmin to produce caeruloplasmin.
  - Caeruloplasmin is excreted into the plasma forming over 90% of plasma copper.
  - Copper is lost from the body via excretion into bile.
  - Both production of caeruloplasmin and biliary excretion of copper require the protein ATP7B.

- Wilson's disease is a rare autosomal recessive disease caused by several mutations of the ATP7B gene.
- Causes accumulation of copper in the liver, brain (basal ganglia) and cornea.

CLINICAL PRESENTATION

- History:
  - Symptoms in children:
    - Variety of hepatic problems:
      o Asymptomatic abnormal LFTs.
      o Acute hepatitis/fulminant hepatic failure.
      o Chronic liver disease.
  - Symptoms in young adults:
    - Neurological symptoms: tremor, dysarthria, dyskinesia.
    - Psychiatric symptoms: depression, phobias, compulsive behaviour.
  - Symptoms of both liver and neurological involvement may be present.
  - Other presentations include:
    - Gallstones secondary to recurrent haemolysis.
    - Renal disease: e.g. Fanconi's syndrome (disease of proximal renal tubule leading to loss of bicarbonate, amino acids, glucose and phosphate).
    - Arthritis secondary to copper deposition in synovium.
    - Osteoporosis.
    - Cardiomyopathy.
- Examination:
  - Kayser–Fleischer rings: green/brown pigment deposition around the edge of the cornea at the junction with the sclera.
  - Mixed neurological and hepatic signs.

INVESTIGATIONS

- Blood tests:
  - Elevated transaminases.
  - Low serum caeruloplasmin.
  - Low serum copper.
- Urinary copper excretion:
  - Increased: over 100 mg in 24 hours (normal is <40 mg).
  - Penicillamine challenge: 500 mg 12 hourly for 24 hours.
- Liver biopsy:
  - Increased hepatic copper levels are found.
- Genetic analysis:
  - More than 260 mutations in the ATP7B gene reported so usually only common mutations tested for.

MANAGEMENT

- Penicillamine:
  - Chelating agent which binds to copper and is excreted in the urine.
- Trientine:
  - Increases urine excretion of copper.
- Zinc:
  - Reduces copper absorption and increases faecal excretion.

10.11 HEPATOCELLULAR CARCINOMA

DEFINITION

- Primary malignancy arising from the hepatocytes.

EPIDEMIOLOGY

- Geographical associations:
  - Highest incidence is found in Asia and sub-Saharan Africa.
  - Reflects incidence of hepatitis B (see below).
- More common in men.
- Increased incidence with age – 70% are over 65 years of age.
- Sixth most common cancer worldwide, 18th most common in UK:
  - UK incidence is around 4 per 100,000 population.
- Incidence increasing in UK.

RISK FACTORS/AETIOLOGY

- Cirrhosis of the liver (regardless of cause): 1/3 will develop HCC.
- Viral hepatitis: hepatitis B and C viruses.
- Aflatoxin: toxins produced by certain fungi.
- Androgenic steroids.
- Oral contraceptive pill: weak association.

PATHOPHYSIOLOGY

- Grading:
  - Barcelona Clinic Liver Cancer (BCLC) classification takes into account the number and size of liver nodules, liver function (Child-Pugh score), presence of portal invasion, metastasis and general health.

MICRO-reference

For further information on the Barcelona Clinical Liver Cancer classification, see: http://www.hepatitis.va.gov/provider/guidelines/2009HCC-bclc-staging.asp?backto=provider/guidelines/2009HCC&backtext=Back%20to%202009%20HCC%20Recommendations

---

Gastroenterology

- Metastatic spread:
  - HCC commonly metastasizes to the lungs, bone, brain and the portal vein.

CLINICAL FEATURES

- History:
  - Ascites.
  - Jaundice.
  - Abdominal pain: right hypochondrium.
  - Anorexia/weight loss.
- Examination:
  - Jaundice.
  - Hepatomegaly: liver may be hard and irregular.
  - Stigmata of chronic liver disease (see Section 4.1).

INVESTIGATIONS

- Blood tests:
  - α-Fetoprotein (AFP) may be normal in early disease.
  - LFTs/clotting: deranged due to underlying liver disease/infiltration.
- Imaging:
  - CXR: may show lung metastases.
  - USS: mass/focal liver lesion on a background of chronic liver disease.
    - Raised AFP and a mass of >2 cm is diagnostic.
  - Contrast CT/contrast MRI:
    - Staging.
- Biopsy:
  - Diagnostic in cases where diagnosis is unclear.
  - Avoid in curative disease: risk of tumour seeding in needle tract.

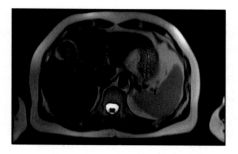

Figure 10.6 MRI showing hepatocellular carcinoma.

MANAGEMENT

- Surgical resection:
  - Used for small (<3 cm) solitary tumours with good liver function (Child-Pugh grade A).
  - High risk of further tumours developing in the remaining liver.
- Liver transplant:
  - Milan criteria used to select appropriate patients (see MICRO-facts box).
  - Beneficial for patients unsuitable for resection owing to advanced liver disease.
- Chemo-embolization (TACE – transcatheter arterial chemo-embolization):
  - Administration of chemotherapy drugs directly to tumour.
- Ablation:
  - Radiofrequency ablation:
    - Ultrasound probe placed into tumour can cause tumour necrosis.
  - Microwave ablation:
    - Microwave probes damage tumour cells using heat.
- Systemic chemotherapy:
  - Sorafanib for Child-Pugh grade A disease.

MICRO-facts

Milan criteria:
  One lesion <5 cm or 3 lesions <3 cm
  No extrahepatic manifestations
  No vascular invasion

PROGNOSIS

- Depends on condition of underlying liver:
  - Stage 0/A – 5-year survival is 40–70%.
  - Stage B – median survival of 20 months after TACE.
  - Stage C (advanced disease) – median survival of 11 months.
  - Stage D (terminal disease) – median survival <3 months.

10.12 METASTATIC LIVER DISEASE

PATHOPHYSIOLOGY

- 90% of liver tumours in Europe are metastatic.
- Common primary cancers at other sites which spread to the liver include the GI tract, breasts, lungs and pancreas.
- Usually there are multiple tumours affecting both lobes of the liver.

CLINICAL FEATURES

- Examination:
  - Hepatomegaly.
  - Ascites.
  - Jaundice.
  - Weight loss.

INVESTIGATIONS

- Blood tests:
  - Deranged LFTs in most patients:
    - Typically raised ALP/γGT.
- Imaging:
  - USS.
  - Contrast CT.
  - Contrast MRI.
- Biopsy:
  - Can provide histological diagnosis.

MANAGEMENT

- If there is not a known primary tumour, then investigations should be focused on searching for it:
  - CT chest/abdomen/pelvis.
- Management of liver metastases depends on the number lesions and the origin of the tumour:
  - Down-staging chemotherapy followed by surgery can lead to prolonged survival in colorectal cancer.
  - Tumours such as breast cancer often respond well to chemotherapy/ hormonal therapy.
  - Liver metastases from aggressive tumours such as lung, pancreas and stomach respond poorly to chemotherapy.
  - Multiple lesions/advanced primary cancer may mean any intervention in the liver is futile.

PROGNOSIS

- Dependent on the primary tumour/extent and number of metastases.

10.13 BUDD–CHIARI SYNDROME

DEFINITION

- Occlusion of hepatic vein causing obstruction of venous outflow from the liver.

EPIDEMIOLOGY

- The incidence is estimated at around 1 case per million population per year.

AETIOLOGY

- Haematology:
  - Hypercoagulable states: polycythaemia vera, antiphospholipid syndrome, leukaemia etc.
- Reduction in blood flow:
  - Abnormal vena cava – webs.
  - Right renal/adrenal tumours.
  - HCC.
- Pregnancy.
- Medications: oral contraceptive pill, hormone replacement therapy.
- Trauma.
- Chronic inflammation: IBD, systemic lupus erythematosus.

CLINICAL FEATURES

- Acute presentation:
  - Abdominal pain with tender liver.
  - Nausea and vomiting.
  - Hepatomegaly.
  - Ascites.
  - Jaundice.
- Chronic presentation:
  - Ascites.
  - Mild jaundice.
  - Hepatomegaly ± splenomegaly.

INVESTIGATIONS

- Blood tests:
  - LFTs: may be normal or mildly elevated.
  - FBC, thrombophilia screen, JAK2 analysis (for underlying clotting/myeloproliferative disorders).
- Ascitic fluid analysis: high protein content.
- Histology: centrilobular congestion, haemorrhage, fibrosis.
- Imaging:
  - USS Doppler: hepatic vein occlusion.
  - CT/MRI: enlarged caudate lobe and/or hepatic vein occlusion.
  - Venography: if diagnosis remains uncertain or for treatment.

MANAGEMENT

- Identification and treatment of cause.
- Anticoagulation.
- Thrombolysis: for acute disease, local or systemic.
- Management of ascites: diuretics, fluid and salt restriction.
- Decompression:
  - Angioplasty ± stent for acute disease.
  - Transjugular intrahepatic portosystemic shunts (TIPS):
    - A shunt is created between the portal and systemic vasculature.
- Transplant:
  - For chronic Budd–Chiari syndrome.
  - Followed by lifelong anticoagulation to prevent recurrence.

COMPLICATIONS

- Portal hypertension.
- Variceal haemorrhage.
- Other complications of hypercoagulability.

10.14 VENO-OCCLUSIVE DISEASE

DEFINITION

- Occlusion of terminal hepatic venules, hepatic sinusoids.
- Also known as sinusoidal obstruction syndrome.

EPIDEMIOLOGY

- Rare but affects a significant proportion of bone marrow transplant patients.

AETIOLOGY

- Post ingestion of some herbal teas: pyrrolizidine alkaloids.
- Post chemotherapy and total body irradiation prior to bone marrow transplant.
- Rare hereditary variant.
- Cyclophosphamide.

PATHOLOGY

- Toxic agents damage hepatic vein endothelium.
- Causes occlusion of the small veins and hence a reduction in hepatic blood flow.

CLINICAL FEATURES

- Similar to Budd–Chiari syndrome.
- Weight gain: secondary to renal failure.

- Ascites.
- Tender hepatomegaly.
- Raised bilirubin.

INVESTIGATIONS

- Blood tests:
  - LFTs: raised bilirubin.
- Imaging:
  - USS Doppler/CT/MRI: exclude hepatic vein occlusion, biliary disease.
- Transjugular liver biopsy and measurement of hepatic venous pressure gradient:
  - Gradient of >10 mmHg suggestive of veno-occlusive disease.
  - Biopsy shows occlusion of sinusoids/venules.

MANAGEMENT

- Mainly supportive as condition often resolves after 2–3 weeks:
  - Ascites: diuretics/paracentesis.
  - TIPS for refractory ascites but long-term outcome usually poor.
  - Liver transplant can be considered depending on comorbidity.

10.15 PORTAL VEIN THROMBOSIS

DEFINITION

- Thrombosis of the portal vein that results in a reduction in hepatic blood flow and portal hypertension.

AETIOLOGY

- Hypercoagulable states: e.g. protein C or S deficiency, Factor V Leiden mutation.
- Inflammatory condition: e.g. IBD, pancreatitis.
- Infections: e.g. appendicitis, cholecystitis, cholangitis, diverticulitis.
- Impaired flow: e.g. cirrhosis, pancreatic cancer, HCC.
- Complications of therapy: splenectomy, hepatobiliary surgery, peritoneal dialysis.

PATHOLOGY

- Thrombosis can be partial or complete.
- Liver function usually unaffected due to compensatory mechanisms:
  - Increased arterial perfusion.
  - Venous collaterals: oesophageal varices etc.

CLINICAL FEATURES

- Often asymptomatic.
- Acute onset (uncommon):
  - Abdominal pain, nausea, diarrhoea: due involvement of mesenteric veins.
  - Significant ascites is rare.
  - Splenomegaly.
- Chronic onset (common):
  - Usually presents with complications: e.g. variceal bleeding, ascites.
  - Splenomegaly/pancytopenia.

INVESTIGATIONS

- Blood tests:
  - LFTs usually normal unless there is an underlying liver condition.
  - D-dimer levels may be raised.
  - Thrombophilia screen.
- Imaging:
  - USS: thrombus in portal vein.
  - USS Doppler: reduction in portal vein flow.
  - CT with contrast: filling defect in portal vein.
  - Endoscopic ultrasound: if abdominal USS is difficult due to overlying bowel gas or obesity and contrast CT not possible owing to renal failure.

MANAGEMENT

- Treat upper GI bleed (see Section 1.3).
- Anticoagulation: for acute thrombosis prevents progression of thrombosis.
- Thrombolysis for acute portal vein thrombosis.
- TIPS: technically difficult owing to portal vein thrombosis.
- Shunt surgery.

PROGNOSIS

- Prognosis is good although reduced if cirrhosis coexists.
- Mortality rate is less than 10%.

MICRO-case

A 58-year-old man presents to you in a GP surgery complaining of lethargy, polydipsia and polyuria. His symptoms have been progressing for the last few months. On further questioning he admits to suffering from erectile dysfunction and says he has had joint pains for a number of years.

continued...

continued...

Urinalysis shows glycosuria but is otherwise normal. A fasting blood test is arranged to assess the patient's blood glucose and to find a cause for his symptoms.

Blood test results show a fasting blood glucose level of 13.5 mmol/L. The patient is also noted to have raised ferritin and serum iron levels. Liver functions tests are normal.

Genetic analysis is arranged for the patient that shows a homozygous mutation in the HFE gene and a diagnosis of haemochromatosis is made. Further endocrine investigations show hypogonadism with reduced testosterone levels. The patient is referred to endocrinology for testosterone replacement to reduce the risk of osteoporosis secondary to hypogonadism and liver disease. An echocardiograph is arranged to assess cardiac function.

An assessment is made of the patient's liver function, as normal liver function tests do not rule out liver disease. An abdominal ultrasound scan is performed followed by a liver biopsy to assess the liver for cirrhosis. α-Fetoprotein (AFP) levels are checked to screen for hepatocellular carcinoma.

Venesection is commenced and 500 mL of blood is removed. The patient is advised this will be repeated each week until blood tests have normalized.

Key points:

- Haemochromatosis is a pathological build up of iron in a range of tissues.
- It often presents late once the build up of iron has caused damage to tissues.
- Males present earlier than females as menstruation has a protective effect.
- Erectile dysfunction, diabetes mellitus and arthropathy can all be seen, as in this patient.
- Treatment is with venesection to remove iron from the body. Often 30–40 units are removed over a period of months to return iron levels to normal.
- Genetic counselling is important to educate patients and their families.
- Diabetes in haemochromatosis is due to pancreatic failure rather than insulin resistance so metformin is of limited use.

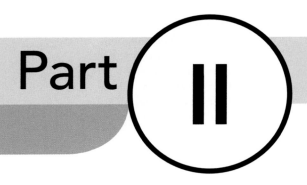

Part II

Self-assessment

Gastroenterology

Questions

COMMON UPPER GI PRESENTATIONS: EMQ

For each of the following clinical scenarios, all of which focus on oesophageal presentations, please choose the most appropriate diagnosis. Each option can be used once, more than once or not at all.

1) Achalasia
2) Foreign body
3) Oesophageal carcinoma
4) Oesophageal spasm
5) Oesophageal stricture
6) Oesophageal web
7) Oesophagitis
8) Pharyngeal carcinoma
9) Pharyngeal pouch
10) Stroke

Question 1

A 55-year-old woman presents with a history of intermittent dysphagia associated with central chest pain. Ischaemic heart disease is considered but excluded by normal cardiac investigations. What is the most likely diagnosis?

Question 2

A 64-year-old man presents with a progressive history of dysphagia to solids over the previous 3 months. He is a lifelong smoker, smoking around 30 cigarettes per day. Upon further questioning he reveals he has unintentionally lost 2 stone over a similar time frame. What is the most likely diagnosis?

Question 3

A 75-year-old man presents with a fever, cough and pleuritic chest pain. He is found to have pneumonia. Upon questioning he reveals he has been having difficulty swallowing and has been regurgitating food soon after eating. What is the most likely diagnosis?

COMMON UPPER GI PRESENTATIONS: SBA

For the following clinical scenario, please select the single best answer from the list below.

1) Hyperchloraemic acidosis with hyperkalaemia
2) Hyperchloraemic acidosis with hypokalaemia
3) Hypochloraemic acidosis with hyperkalaemia
4) Hypochloraemic alkalosis with hyperkalaemia
5) Hypochloraemic alkalosis with hypokalaemia

Question 4

A 65-year-old woman patient is admitted with profuse vomiting of unknown cause. As part of her initial investigations several biochemical tests are undertaken. Of the electrolyte imbalances listed above, which is most likely to be found in this patient?

COMMON SMALL BOWEL PRESENTATIONS: EMQ

For each of the following clinical scenarios, all of which focus on vitamin deficiencies, please choose the correct deficiency. Each option may be used once, more than once or not at all.

1) Vitamin A
2) Vitamin B_1
3) Vitamin B_6
4) Vitamin B_{12}
5) Vitamin C
6) Vitamin D
7) Vitamin E
8) Vitamin K

Question 5

A 56-year-old man is admitted to the ward after being found wandering in the street by a neighbour. There is a collateral history suggesting long-term alcohol misuse. The patient is unsteady on his feet and appears confused. Deficiency of which vitamin could account for this patient's symptoms?

Question 6

A 59-year-old woman with a long history of autoimmune hepatitis is admitted to the ward with a deterioration in her condition. She is noted to have widespread bruises and bleeds more than expected after venepuncture. Deficiency of which vitamin is responsible for this patient's problems?

Question 7

Four years after a terminal ileal resection for Crohn's disease, a patient visits his or her GP with worsening tiredness and vague neurological symptoms. The patient has missed numerous follow-up appointments. Blood tests show a megaloblastic anaemia. Deficiency of which vitamin is responsible for this patient's problems?

COMMON SMALL BOWEL PRESENTATIONS: SBA

For the following clinical scenario, please choose the most appropriate answer from the list below. Select the best single answer, each option may be used once only.

1) Aspiration
2) Diarrhoea
3) Hyperglycaemia
4) Oesophagitis
5) Re-feeding syndrome

Question 8

A malnourished patient is admitted to the ward and the decision is made that artificial nutrition is needed. The consultant asks you as the junior doctor to monitor the patient's phosphate, potassium and magnesium levels. Which of the complications listed is the consultant concerned about?

COMMON COLONIC PRESENTATIONS: EMQ

For each of the following clinical scenarios, all of which focus on lower gastrointestinal/colonic presentations, please choose the most appropriate diagnosis. Each option can be used once, more than once or nor at all.

1) Acute appendicitis
2) Acute diverticulitis
3) Acute sigmoid volvulus
4) Chronic pancreatitis
5) Coeliac disease
6) Colorectal cancer
7) Irritable bowel syndrome
8) Meckel's diverticulitis
9) Peptic ulcer disease
10) Pernicious anaemia

Question 9

A 68-year-old farmer was referred by his GP with an 8-week history of altered bowel habit, weight loss, rectal bleeding and intermittent crampy lower abdominal pain. His blood indices showed haemoglobin (Hb) 101 g/L, mean cell volume (MCV) 76 fl, white cell count (WCC) 4.9×10^9/L, platelets (Plts) 254×10^9/L and ferritin 12 ng/mL. What is the most likely diagnosis from the above list?

Question 10

A 21-year-old woman visits her GP with a 5-month history of general malaise. She further reports difficulty in gaining weight but denies any menstrual disturbance (particularly heavy periods). There is no recent change in her bowel habit although she has always had loose motions. She otherwise denies any symptoms of dyspepsia, dysphagia or early satiety. There is no family history of colorectal cancer. Initial blood screening reveals Hb 98 g/L, MCV 69 fl, WCC 3.9×10^9/L, Plts 231×10^9/L, C-reactive protein (CRP) 6 mg/L,

Self-assessment

erythrocyte sedimentation rate (ESR) 11 mm/hr, tissue transglutaminase (tTG) 150 with a positive endomysial antibody (EMA). What is the most likely diagnosis from the above list?

Question 11

A 62-year-old mechanic with osteoarthritis and hypertension attends the ED with two episodes of haematemesis and epigastric pain. He is haemodynamically stable. His medications include paracetamol, diclofenac and amlodipine. What is the most likely diagnosis from the above list?

COMMON COLONIC PRESENTATIONS: SBA

For the following clinical scenario, please select the single best answer from the list below.

1) Colonoscopy
2) CT angiogram ± embolization
3) OGD (oesophago-gastro-duodenoscopy)
4) Small bowel capsule endoscopy
5) Tc-RBC scan (technetium labelling red blood cell scan)

Question 12

You are called to see a 28-year-old fit and well amateur boxer in the ED. The patient is pale with HR 133/min, BP 100/60, RR 25/min, O_2 saturations, 98% on air. He has had three episodes of fresh rectal bleeding for the past 8 hours. He feels nauseated and exhausted. While you are cannulating the patient, he suddenly collapses with subsequent BP 60 systolic. What would be the next best investigation after initial resuscitation?

COMMON LIVER PRESENTATIONS: EMQ

1) Alcoholic hepatitis
2) Autoimmune hepatitis
3) Drug-induced hepatitis
4) Gallstones
5) Gilbert's syndrome
6) Pancreatic carcinoma
7) Pernicious anaemia
8) Primary biliary cirrhosis (PBC)
9) Sickle cell anaemia
10) Viral hepatitis

Question 13

You are a junior doctor working in the ED. A 57-year-old woman presents with a 2-day history of nausea and intermittent, severe epigastric, colicky pain which is radiating to her back. Upon examination you notice yellowing of her sclera and epigastric tenderness. Her LFTs show a bilirubin of 65 µmol/L, an ALP of 210 IU/L and a γGT of 232 IU/L. Which of the above conditions is the patient likely to be suffering from?

Question 14

A 22-year-old medical student presents to her GP complaining of 2 weeks of flu-like symptoms. On inspection, she appears jaundiced and has tender hepatomegaly. She has recently been to Southeast Asia on her medical elective and admits to having drunk some of the water while there. LFTs show a raised ALT of 810 IU/L, a bilirubin of 80 μmol/L and a γGT of 120 IU/L. What is the most likely diagnosis?

Question 15

You are working on a gastroenterology ward when a 48-year-old woman is referred to you from her GP. Over the past 18 months, she has been suffering from pruritis which has progressively worsened. Over the past few days, she has become jaundiced. There is no history of drug or alcohol abuse, and she has no recent history of foreign travel. She has a past history of autoimmune thyroid disease. On admission, her LFTs show:

ALT: 96 IU/L	Bilirubin: 68 μmol/L
ALP: 514 IU/L	Albumin: 26 g/L
γGT: 236 IU/L	

What do you suspect is the cause of her symptoms?

COMMON LIVER PRESENTATIONS: SBA

Question 16

You are a junior doctor working in the ED. A 62-year-old man presents suffering from acute alcohol withdrawal. You carry out your initial assessment and administer chlordiazepoxide. Which of the following medications would you also give to ensure that the patient does not begin to suffer the side effects of thiamine deficiency?

1) Acamprosate
2) Diazepam
3) Disulfiram
4) Naltrexone
5) Pabrinex

OESOPHAGUS: EMQ

For each of the following clinical scenarios, all of which focus on oesophageal presentations, please choose the most appropriate diagnosis. Each option can be used once, more than once or not at all.

1) Achalasia
2) Barrett's oesophagus
3) Tracheal-oesophageal fistula
4) Candidiasis
5) Eosinophilic oesophagitis
6) Gastric volvulus
7) Gastro-oesophageal reflux disease (GORD)
8) Oesophageal cancer
9) Pharyngeal pouch

Self-assessment

Question 17

A 28-year-old teacher has been complaining of heartburn and early morning hoarseness for the last 2 months. He denies any recent weight loss, dysphagia or early satiety. During the consultation, he admits to drinking 4 pints of lager every evening. General examination was unremarkable apart from a body mass index (BMI) of 33. What is the most likely diagnosis?

Question 18

A 45-year-old woman is referred to the gastroenterology clinic by her GP with a 3-month history of ongoing weight loss with intermittent dysphagia to both solids and liquids. Her blood tests including full blood count (FBC), urea and electrolytes (U&E), LFTs and CRP were normal. Her upper GI endoscopy together with oesophageal and duodenal biopsies were normal. Subsequent oesophageal manometry showed low amplitude, non-propagating contractions with failure of the lower oesophageal sphincter (LOS) to relax on swallowing. What is the most likely diagnosis?

Question 19

A 72-year-old retired electrician with a known history of long segment Barrett's oesophagus was referred by his own GP with progressive dysphagia to solid food over the past 2 months and a recent history of 1 stone of weight loss. He has been having difficulty swallowing liquid for the past week. What is the most likely diagnosis from the above list?

OESOPHAGUS: SBA

For the following clinical scenario, please select the single best answer from the list below.

1) All of the options
2) Avoidance of late evening meals
3) Smoking cessation
4) Trial of a proton pump inhibitor (PPI)
5) Weight loss

Question 20

A 32-year-old lorry driver attends your clinic with a 2-month history of intermittent retrosternal burning sensation especially at night. He does not report weight loss, dysphagia or early satiety symptoms. He is a current smoker with a BMI of 32. What is your management plan?

For the following clinical scenario, please select the single best answer from the list below.

1) Achalasia
2) Barrett's oesophagus
3) Eosinophilic oesophagitis
4) Gastro-oesophageal reflux disease (GORD)
5) Oesophageal spasm

Question 21

A 26-year-old yoga instructor presents with intermittent regurgitation, heartburn and dysphagia to solids and liquids. There is no history of weight loss or early satiety. She is only on the oral contraceptive pill. Gastroscopy including oesophageal biopsies is normal. Barium swallow shows multiple simultaneous oesophageal contractions with poor propulsion of the food bolus. What is the likely diagnosis?

STOMACH AND DUODENUM: EMQ

For each of the following clinical scenarios, all of which focus upon disorders of the stomach and duodenum, please choose the most relevant intervention. Each option can be used once, more than once or not at all.

1) Antacids
2) Domperidone
3) Endoscopic haemostatic therapy
4) Endoscopic mucosal resection (EMR)
5) Gastrectomy
6) Gastric bypass surgery
7) *Helicobacter pylori* eradication therapy
8) H_2 receptor antagonist
9) Proton pump inhibitor (PPI)
10) Vitamin B_{12} injections

Question 22

You are a junior doctor on the gastroenterology ward. You are asked to clerk in a 36-year-old man suffering from recurrent nausea and vomiting over the last few months. He has lost 6 kg in weight. He has a past history of poorly controlled diabetes mellitus. Examination is normal apart from a succussion splash. He goes on to have a normal gastroscopy although there was a considerable gastric residue. Which of the above treatment options will be likely to benefit the patient?

Question 23

You are a junior doctor on the gastroenterology ward. You are asked to see a 45-year-old man who has been admitted with a 1-month history of upper abdominal pain. He had a myocardial infarction 6 weeks earlier. He has suddenly begun to vomit fresh blood. Which treatment intervention should be considered next?

Question 24

You are a junior doctor in the gastroenterology team. A 78-year-old man has recently been admitted with a long-standing history of epigastric pain. His wife has commented that he has also lost weight. An OGD shows a 1.5 cm carcinoma of the gastric body which is confirmed subsequently by histology. Further staging investigations with CT, EUS and PET scanning shows the cancer is confined to the mucosa of the stomach. Which of the above treatments is most appropriate for this patient?

STOMACH AND DUODENUM: SBA

For each of the following questions, please choose the most appropriate answer from the set of options given. Select the best single answer, each option may be used once only.

Question 25

You are a junior doctor working at a primary care practice when a 74-year-old woman comes into your clinic presenting with a progressive history of fatigue with shortness of breath. She eats a normal diet. On examination, you notice that the patient appears pale and has fissuring around her mouth, causing you to suspect that she may be suffering from anaemia. Blood tests confirm she is anaemic, with a normal serum iron but a low vitamin B_{12}. Autoantibody tests for anti-gastric parietal cells are negative. A further test is ordered to confirm the diagnosis. Which confirmatory test would verify your diagnosis?

1) Barium meal
2) Schilling test
3) Thyroid antibodies
4) Upper GI endoscopy
5) Urea breath test

Question 26

Which of these histological subgroups of gastric cancer accounts for 90% of all gastric cancers?

1) Adenocarcinoma
2) Carcinoid tumour
3) GIST
4) Lymphoma
5) Squamous

Question 27

A 74-year-old woman presents with a 3-month history of worsening vomiting and weight loss of 2 stone. She has angina and COPD with an exercise tolerance of 50 yards on the flat. She is referred for a gastroscopy which shows a tumour of her distal stomach, obstructing the pylorus. Urgent CT shows liver metastases. Given the above information, what would be the next most appropriate step in this patient's management?

1) Endoscopic mucosal resection (EMR)
2) Gastrectomy
3) Gastric bypass
4) Pyloric stenting
5) Radiotherapy

THE SMALL BOWEL: EMQs

EMQ 1

For each of the following clinical scenarios, all of which focus on small bowel diseases, please choose the most likely diagnosis. Each option can be used once, more than once or not at all.

1) Clostridium difficle infection
2) Coeliac disease
3) Lactose intolerance
4) Rotavirus infection
5) Small bowel adenocarcinoma
6) Small bowel carcinoid tumour
7) Small bowel lymphoma
8) Small intestinal bacterial overgrowth
9) Vibrio cholerae infection
10) Whipple's disease

Question 28

A 52-year-old woman presents with a long history of abdominal bloating with occasional diarrhoea. Recently her symptoms have been getting worse with increasing fatigue. Upon further questioning she admits her stools can be difficult to flush. Her past medical history includes type 1 diabetes mellitus and hyperthyroidism. Her blood tests show that she is mildly anaemic, with low iron and folic acid levels but normal B_{12} levels. From the options listed above, what is the likely underlying disease?

Question 29

A 48-year-old bricklayer is seen in the ED with dyspnoea and diarrhoea. On examination, his face is flushed and his BP is low. He admits he has had progressive, intermittent right-sided abdominal discomfort for several months but didn't want to take time off work to see his GP. His weight has recently dropped by 4 kg but he puts this down to stress. From the options listed above, what is the likely underlying disease?

Question 30

A 23-year-old Asian woman visits your GP surgery. She tells you that she has an embarrassing problem with flatulence and loud rumbling sounds from the stomach over recent months. She has a history of abdominal bloating for which she has seen you several times. More recently the symptoms have been accompanied by diarrhoea. From the options listed above, what is the likely underlying disease?

EMQ 2

For each of the following scenarios, please choose the most likely causative organism. Each option can be used once, more than once or not at all.

1) *Bacillus cereus*
2) *Campylobacter* spp.
3) *Clostridium difficile*
4) *Escherichia coli*

5) *Salmonella* spp.
6) *Shigella* spp.
7) *Staphylococcus aureus*
8) *Vibrio cholerae*

Question 31

Three hours after eating at a birthday party, a 9-year-old boy begins vomiting and complains of abdominal pain and subsequently develops diarrhoea. His symptoms resolve within a day and at school on Monday it transpires that three other children who attended the same party had similar symptoms. What is the likely causative organism?

Question 32

A 53-year-old man develops profuse diarrhoea with vomiting 2 days after going out for a meal with his family. His symptoms clear up 5 days later with only supportive treatment needed. Several weeks later he develops weakness, which begins in his legs. He is subsequently diagnosed with Guillain–Barré syndrome. What is the likely causative organism?

Question 33

An 84-year-old man is admitted to the ED with severe diarrhoea and dehydration. His wife tells you he recently had a course of antibiotics for a urinary tract infection (UTI). What is the likely causative organism?

THE SMALL BOWEL: SBA

For the following question, please choose the single most appropriate answer from the options below.

1) CCK (cholecystokinin)
2) Gastrin
3) GIP (glucose-dependent insulinotropic peptide)

4) Secretin
5) Somatostatin

Question 34

This hormone, released in response to amino acids in the small intestine, stimulates pancreatic enzyme release and gallbladder contraction. Which of the above hormones does this description relate to?

For the following question, please choose the single most appropriate answer from the options below.

1) EMA
2) HLA
3) IELs
4) IgA
5) tTG

Question 35

Which of the above is the first-line immunological investigation for coeliac disease?

For the following question, please choose the single most appropriate answer from the options below.

1) Coeliac disease
2) Lactose intolerance
3) Small bowel lymphoma
4) Small intestinal bacterial overgrowth
5) Whipple's disease

Question 36

A 45-year-old man is seen in an outpatient clinic after being referred by his GP. He has a long history of abdominal bloating and diarrhoea, which can be difficult to flush away. There is no association with any types of food. He has recently been feeling increasingly tired. Blood tests show a macrocytic anaemia, negative tTG and a hydrogen breath test is positive. What is the likely diagnosis?

COLORECTAL DISEASE: EMQs

EMQ 1

For each of the following clinical scenarios, all of which focus on lower gastrointestinal/colonic presentations, please choose the most appropriate diagnosis. Each option can be used once, more than once or not at all.

1) Acute diverticulitis
2) Benign ovarian cyst
3) Chronic constipation
4) Chronic fatigue syndrome
5) Coeliac disease
6) Inflammatory bowel disease
7) Irritable bowel syndrome (constipation predominant)
8) Irritable bowel syndrome (diarrhoea predominant)
9) Prostatitis
10) Small bowel obstruction

Question 37

A 66-year-old taxi driver with a long history of chronic intermittent constipation was admitted to the ED following 12 hours of intermittent rectal bleeding, abdominal pain and low-grade fever. He did not report any recent weight loss or change in bowel habit prior to this current event. On examination, he was haemodynamically stable with a tender abdomen over the left iliac fossa. There was no palpable underlying mass. What is the most likely diagnosis from the above list?

Question 38

A 19-year-old medical student attended her GP with a 3-month history of feeling generally 'under the weather' with associated intermittent right iliac fossa pain and 1 stone of weight loss. On examination, she was haemodynamically stable with tenderness over the right iliac fossa. Blood test results showed Hb 115 g/L, MCV 85 fl, Plts 518 × 10⁹/L, WCC 9.1 × 10⁹/L, ferritin 88 ng/mL, tTG and EMA negative, ESR 28 mm/hr, CRP 23 mg/L, normal LFT and normal U&E. Her pregnancy test was also negative. What is the most likely diagnosis from the above list?

Question 39

A 35-year-old charity worker presented to her GP with a 3-year history of intermittent constipation, bloating and abdominal pain. She reported symptom improvement post-defecation. She had put on several kilograms in weight. She denied any nocturnal symptoms of abdominal pain or bloating. General examination was unremarkable. Screening bloods including FBC, U&E, LFT, thyroid function tests (TFTs), CRP, ESR and coeliac serology were normal. What is the most likely diagnosis from the list above?

EMQ 2

For each of the following clinical scenarios, all of which focus on colonic presentations, please choose the most appropriate treatment. Each option can be used once, more than once or not at all.

1) Budesonide
2) Ciclosporin
3) Infliximab
4) Intravenous (IV) antibiotics
5) IV hydrocortisone
6) Methotrexate
7) Oral fluid therapy
8) Surgery
9) Prucalopride
10) Thiopurines

Question 40

A 23-year-old librarian with known ulcerative colitis attends the ED with a 3-week history of worsening bloody diarrhoea. He has been opening his bowels up to 12 times daily for the past 2 days and he reports rectal bleeding mixed in with the stool. On examination, his vital signs are BP 120/78, HR 92/minute, RR 15/minute, temperature 37.6°C. His abdomen is mildly tender over the left iliac fossa but no guarding is felt. Initial blood results show Hb 101 g/L, MCV 81 fl, WCC 11.2 × 10⁹/L, CRP 49 mg/L. Following initial investigations, what would be the most appropriate therapy at this stage?

Question 41

A 45-year-old man with known Crohn's colitis has had two episodes of the disease flaring up that required steroids therapy over the last year. What would be the first-line maintenance therapy?

Question 42

A 21-year-old woman with a history of chronic constipation since her early teenage years has had worsening of her symptoms over the past year. She is already on maximum dose therapy with sodium docusate and senna. What would be the next best option?

COLORECTAL DISEASE: SBAs

SBA 1

For the following clinical scenario, please select the single best answer from the list below.

1) CA-125
2) CEA
3) Coeliac serology
4) CRP
5) FBC

Question 43

A 46-year-old woman with a long history of lower abdominal pain and an erratic bowel habit is referred to you with typical IBS symptoms as per the Rome III criteria. Which of the above investigations is not necessary?

SBA 2

For the following clinical scenario, please select the single best answer from the list below.

1) Bowel obstruction
2) Colorectal cancer
3) Chronic diverticular disease
4) Ischaemic colitis
5) Melanosis coli

Question 44

A 76-year-old retired pilot with known ischaemic heart disease and paroxysmal atrial fibrillation attended the ED with left iliac fossa pain. In addition, he revealed that he had been having small but frequent passage of maroon-coloured loose stools for the past 24 hours. His regular medications included digoxin, spironolactone, bendroflumethiazide, aspirin, bisoprolol and lisinopril. He was haemodynamically stable and general abdominal examination revealed slight tenderness. Initial blood test results showed raised serum lactate and neutrophil count. Abdominal X-ray (AXR) revealed normal small and large bowel diameters with unremarkable intraluminal gas distribution; there were however signs of mucosal thickening (thumb-printing) in the left colon. What is the likely diagnosis?

PANCREATOBILIARY DISEASE: EMQ

For each of the following clinical scenarios, please choose the correct clinical intervention. Each option may be used once, more than once or not at all.

1) Biliary drainage
2) Chemotherapy
3) Dissolution therapy
4) ERCP
5) Extracorporeal shock wave lithotripsy
6) IV fluids
7) Laparoscopic cholecystectomy
8) Pancreaticoduodenectomy
9) Radiotherapy
10) Surgical resection with partial hepatectomy

Question 45

You are a junior doctor working on a gastroenterology ward when a 48-year-old overweight woman is admitted with severe right upper quadrant pain and fever which is spreading around her back. She is Murphy's sign positive. On looking through her old notes, you discover that she suffers from type 2 diabetes mellitus. What is the definitive treatment for this woman's condition?

Question 46

You are working in the ED when you are asked to see a 65-year-old man with sudden-onset epigastric pain which is radiating to his back. On examination, you notice that there appears to be some bruising around the umbilical region. His wife admits that the patient has been drinking heavily for several months. What immediate treatment would you administer?

Question 47

You are on the gastroenterology ward when a 72-year-old man arrives, having been referred to you by his GP. The patient is clearly jaundiced and has begun to experience epigastric pain. He reports having lost a significant amount of weight over the past 2 months. A CT scan is done, which shows carcinoma of the head of the pancreas. The tumour appears localized and there are no visible metastases. What definitive treatment option would you recommend?

PANCREATOBILIARY DISEASE: SBA

For each of the following clinical scenarios, please choose the single most appropriate answer from the options given.

Question 48

You are working on a palliative care ward when an 87-year-old man with known end-stage pancreatic carcinoma is admitted. During your examination of the patient, you notice that his left calf appears swollen and red. His wife comments that she noticed swelling in his right leg a few days before his admission. Which of the following eponymous signs is this patient exhibiting?

1) Courvoisier's sign
2) Cullen's sign
3) Grey Turner's sign
4) Murphy's sign
5) Trousseau's sign

Question 49

Which histological subgroup of gallbladder cancer accounts for approximately 85% of all cases?

1) Adenocarcinoma
2) Neuroendocrine tumour
3) Sarcoma
4) Small cell carcinoma
5) Squamous cell carcinoma

Question 50

Which one of the substances secreted by the pancreas is stored in an inactivated form?

1) Amylase
2) Bicarbonate ions
3) Insulin
4) Lipase
5) Proteolytic enzymes

LIVER DISEASE: EMQs

EMQ 1

For each of the following clinical scenarios, please choose the correct diagnosis. Each option can be used once, more than once or not at all.

1) Alcohol-related liver disease
2) Autoimmune hepatitis
3) Hepatitis A
4) Hepatitis B
5) Hepatitis C
6) Hepatitis E
7) Hereditary haemochromatosis
8) Primary biliary cirrhosis (PBC)
9) Primary sclerosing cholangitis (PSC)
10) Wilson's disease

Question 51

You are working as a junior doctor on a gastroenterology ward when you are asked to clerk in a patient who has been referred to the hospital by his GP.

The patient is a 52-year-old man who has been experiencing pain in the right upper quadrant of his abdomen over the past month. More recently he has begun to suffer from a widespread itching sensation, and his wife claims that he has lost weight. On looking through the patient's notes, you discover that he has a long-standing history of ulcerative colitis for which he is taking oral mesalazine. Subsequent investigations show the patient to be P-ANCA positive. What do you suspect his diagnosis to be at this stage?

Question 52

A 22-year-old woman presents to your clinic complaining of a 5-day history of nausea and abdominal pain. The patient tells you that 2 weeks earlier she returned from a holiday to Southeast Asia, where she stayed in hostels and ate a lot of the local cuisine. She had inoculations against hepatitis A before her holiday. On examination, you notice that the patient is feverish, and her sclerae appear jaundiced. What is the most likely diagnosis?

Question 53

You are working in a gastroenterology clinic when a 38-year-old woman comes to see you with a 3-week history of right upper abdominal pain, nausea and fatigue. On further questioning, she reveals that she has also been experiencing pain in her joints. On examination, you note that the patient appears mildly jaundiced. Blood tests show that she is ANA-positive. Which condition is she likely to be suffering from?

EMQ 2

For the following clinical scenarios, please choose the correct diagnosis. Each option can be used once, more than once or not at all.

1) Alcoholic liver disease (ALD)
2) Drug-induced hepatitis
3) Hepatitis B
4) Hepatitis C
5) Hepatocellular carcinoma (HCC)
6) Hereditary haemochromatosis
7) Metastatic liver disease
8) Non-alcoholic fatty liver disease (NAFLD)
9) Primary biliary cirrhosis (PBC)
10) Wilson's disease

Question 54

A 68-year-old man of Malawian origin presents with right upper quadrant pain, jaundice and weight loss. On examination, the liver is hard and irregular. Upon imaging, he is found to have a liver tumour. What is the most likely co-existing condition?

Question 55

An 81-year-old woman presents with a 2-week history of jaundice and weight loss. Upon examination, she is found to have ascites and hepatomegaly. She has no history of liver problems. An ultrasound scan of the liver finds multiple masses within the liver parenchyma. What is the most likely diagnosis?

Question 56

A 54-year-old man who has previously been fit and well presents to you with erectile dysfunction, polydipsia and knee pain. He has recently been feeling increasingly depressed. He remembers his grandfather had a similar condition many years ago. What is the likely diagnosis?

LIVER DISEASE: SBA

For each of the following questions, please choose the most appropriate answer from the options given. Select the single best answer.

Question 57

You are asked to perform venepuncture on a 19-year-old medical student, in order to assess his immunization status following the completion of a hepatitis B vaccination course. Which of the following proteins would you expect to find in the patient's blood to indicate that he has been vaccinated against hepatitis B?

1) Hepatitis B core antigen
2) Hepatitis B envelope antibody
3) Hepatitis B envelope antigen
4) Hepatitis B surface antibody
5) Hepatitis B surface antigen

Question 58

You are working as a junior doctor on a gastroenterology ward when you are asked by the nurses to see a 49-year-old woman who is currently undergoing treatment for primary biliary cirrhosis. The patient is complaining of widespread itching, which she says has been keeping her up at night. On checking her drug chart, you realize that the patient has not been prescribed any symptomatic relief for her pruritis. Which of the following medications would you prescribe for your patient?

1) Cholestyramine
2) Methotrexate
3) Pegylated interferon-α
4) Prednisolone
5) Ursodeoxycholic acid

Question 59

Mallory's hyaline is a histological finding associated most commonly with which disease?

1) Alcoholic liver disease (ALD)
2) Hepatocellular carcinoma (HCC)
3) Hereditary haemochromatosis
4) Non-alcoholic fatty liver disease (NAFLD)
5) Wilson's disease

Self-assessment

Answers

COMMON UPPER GI PRESENTATIONS: EMQ

Answer 1

4) **Oesophageal spasm.** Often presents with non-cardiac chest pain, which can be difficult to distinguish from cardiac causes and may be initially diagnosed as angina. The intermittent nature of the symptoms suggests she is suffering from oesophageal spasm. Another possible diagnosis is achalasia, but this would not be expected to be intermittent and chest pain is not as predominant a feature.

Answer 2

3) **Oesophageal carcinoma.** The progressive nature, history of smoking and weight loss suggest cancer as a diagnosis here. Other progressive causes of dysphagia are less strongly linked to smoking. Another possible cause of these symptoms with this history would be a lung tumour causing external compression of the oesophagus.

Answer 3

9) **Pharyngeal pouch.** This man has aspiration pneumonia. Several of the conditions listed above may cause aspiration pneumonia but the regurgitation, advanced age and male gender suggest that a pharyngeal pouch is the cause of the symptoms.

COMMON UPPER GI PRESENTATIONS: SBA

Answer 4

5) **Hypochloraemic alkalosis with hypokalaemia.** The stomach contains hydrochloric acid (HCl). As such when stomach contents are lost during vomiting, two things happen as a direct result. First, the patient can become alkalotic due to the loss of hydrogen ions. Second, the patient can become hypochloraemic due to the loss of chloride ions. The resulting biochemical imbalance triggers the kidneys to retain more hydrogen ions via an H^+/K^+ exchange pump. As a consequence, more potassium ions are lost and a hypokalaemic state develops. Of the answers listed above 1, 2 and 3 are all acidotic states and therefore can be immediately ruled out. While option 4 is indeed a hypochloraemic alkalosis, there is a high potassium, making this answer incorrect.

COMMON SMALL BOWEL PRESENTATIONS: EMQ

Answer 5

2) **Vitamin B$_1$.** Wernicke's encephalopathy is caused by a deficiency of vitamin B$_1$. It is common in patients who abuse alcohol and presents with a triad of ophthalmoplegia, confusion and ataxia. It is reversible and should be treated with IV vitamin replacement (Pabrinex). For more information, see Section 4.3. It is likely this patient is deficient in other vitamins but it is only vitamin B$_1$ which results in this clinical picture.

Answer 6

8) **Vitamin K.** Vitamin K deficiency results in defects in coagulation as seen in this patient. This is because vitamin K is vital in the production of several clotting factors (II, VII, IX and X). The long history of autoimmune hepatitis in this patient is likely to have resulted in chronic liver failure. This can result in a reduction in bile salt formation leading to a reduction in the absorption of fat-soluble vitamins (including vitamin K). As such, there is a reduction in circulating clotting factors and coagulation defects result. While other vitamins listed are also fat soluble (vitamins A, D and E), deficiencies in these vitamins do not cause problems in coagulation.

Answer 7

4) **Vitamin B$_{12}$.** This patient has a vitamin B$_{12}$ deficiency. Vitamin B$_{12}$ is absorbed in the terminal ileum and if this is surgically removed then the patient requires 3-monthly vitamin B$_{12}$ injections to maintain levels. Body vitamin B$_{12}$ stores will last for a few years, so this patient has only just become deficient, 4 years after the surgery. Vitamin B$_{12}$ deficiency causes a megaloblastic anaemia (leading to this patient's tiredness) and also neurological symptoms. For more detail on vitamin B$_{12}$, see Section 6.5. Other vitamin deficiencies can cause neurological problems (vitamin B6 and vitamin E) but these are not causes of anaemia.

COMMON SMALL BOWEL PRESENTATIONS: SBA

Answer 8

5) **Re-feeding syndrome.** This patient is at risk of re-feeding syndrome. The patient is malnourished and in need of artificial nutrition, so it is likely there has been a period of poor nutritional intake. Resumption of nutrition in patients after a period of poor nutritional intake can cause

re-feeding syndrome. For full details of re-feeding syndrome and artificial nutrition, see Section 2.3. While all the complications listed can occur in patients started on artificial nutrition, levels of phosphate, potassium and magnesium are not affected.

COMMON COLONIC PRESENTATIONS: EMQ

Answer 9

6) **Colorectal cancer.** The low ferritin level and microcytosis suggest iron deficiency. Considering the recent change in bowel habit, weight loss, rectal bleeding as well as the patient's age, lower GI malignancy should be urgently investigated. An 8-week history of intermittent pain together with normal inflammatory markers (WCC, CRP, ESR) make acute diverticulitis, acute appendicitis, acute sigmoid volvulus and Meckel's diverticulitis unlikely diagnoses. Although coeliac disease could be a possibility, rectal bleeding is not a feature of this condition (unless there is secondary small bowel malignancy, which is not included in the above list). Irritable bowel syndrome is not associated with weight loss, iron deficiency anaemia or rectal bleeding. Pernicious anaemia is a chronic macrocytic anaemia due to impaired absorption of vitamin B_{12}. The classic symptoms are weakness, paraesthesia, unsteady gait and painful red tongue. Weight loss may also occur due to anorexia. None of these features are listed in the above case description.

Answer 10

5) **Coeliac disease.** Iron deficiency anaemia in a young woman with a history of poor weight gain is suggestive of coeliac disease (female to male ratio: 3 to 1). Positive tTG and EMA also make coeliac disease diagnosis very likely.

The diagnosis is normally confirmed by upper GI endoscopy and duodenal biopsy (villous atrophy, increased intra-epithelial lymphocytes and crypt hyperplasia).

The duration of this patient's symptoms excludes acute appendicitis, acute diverticulitis, acute sigmoid volvulus and Meckel's diverticulitis. Colorectal cancer is very uncommon in this age group with no family history of colorectal cancer. Although coeliac disease is associated with an increased risk of chronic pancreatitis, specific features of chronic pancreatitis (intermittent attacks of severe abdominal pain especially post-prandially, weight loss, diarrhoea and steatorrhoea due to exocrine insufficiency) have not been described here.

Answer 11

9) **Peptic ulcer disease.** These symptoms are suggestive of upper GI bleeding probably as a result of NSAID use, hence peptic ulcer disease is the most likely diagnosis from the above list.

The pain pattern and haematemesis are not suggestive of acute appendicitis. Upper GI bleeding is not a feature of uncomplicated coeliac disease. Perforated Meckel's diverticulum, acute diverticulitis and colorectal cancer can all present with lower GI bleeding but not upper GI bleeding. Irritable bowel syndrome and chronic pancreatitis do not cause upper GI bleeding. Blood loss can be a cause of iron deficiency anaemia (not pernicious anaemia).

COMMON COLONIC PRESENTATIONS: SBA

Answer 12

3) **OGD.** Tachycardia ± hypotension in an otherwise young and healthy patient is a sign of significant intravascular volume loss secondary to profuse GI bleeding. Due to the high capacity of cardiovascular compensation, hypotension is commonly the last marker of haemodynamic instability in young and fit individuals and clearly indicates critical volume loss. Although the source of bleeding could be distal to the ligament of Treitz (lower GI), an upper GI source of bleeding should first be excluded in this haemodynamically unstable patient due to relative ease of arranging for emergency OGD and high diagnostic yield. Peptic ulcer disease due to regular NSAIDs ± anabolic steroid use is a reasonable causative speculation in this otherwise young and healthy patient but bear in mind that NSAID-induced ulcers can also develop in the lower GI territory.

COMMON LIVER PRESENTATIONS: EMQ

Answer 13

4) **Gallstones.** This woman's LFTs show an obstructive pattern which is suggestive of a stone in the common bile duct. Severe, colicky, epigastric pain radiating to the back is a typical clinical presentation of gallstones. With no apparent history of alcohol abuse or risk-taking behaviours, there is no indication for alcoholic or viral hepatitis. With no provided past medical history of autoimmune disease, clinical suspicion of an autoimmune cause, in the absence of relevant symptoms, should be low (autoimmune hepatitis does not cause severe abdominal pain; if it causes pain, it tends to be more of a constant ache).

Answer 14

10) **Viral hepatitis.** This student is likely to be suffering from hepatitis A, which is endemic to Southeast Asia. Her LFTs show a markedly elevated ALT which is indicative of the liver inflammation caused by acute viral hepatitis. Since her ALT is far more elevated than her γGT, an obstructive cause for her symptoms seems unlikely.

Self-assessment

Answer 15

8) **Primary biliary cirrhosis.** This woman's history shows a chronic picture with symptoms developing over 18 months; her low albumin also suggests chronic disease. Her LFTs indicate an obstructive condition causing secondary liver disease. Considering her gender, history of an autoimmune condition, presentation of chronic pruritis and lack of risk factors for other diseases, primary biliary cirrhosis would be the most likely cause of her symptoms.

COMMON LIVER PRESENTATIONS: SBA

Answer 16

5) **Pabrinex.** IV Pabrinex is given to patients suffering from acute alcohol withdrawal to prevent the onset of Wernicke's encephalopathy. It contains B and C vitamins. Acamprosate and disulfiram are both medications used to increase a patient's chances of remaining abstinent from alcohol. Diazepam is generally used to minimize the symptoms of withdrawal (as is chlordiazepoxide) and naltrexone reduces the psychological effects of alcohol withdrawal on the patient.

OESOPHAGUS: EMQ

Answer 17

7) **Gastro-oesophageal reflux disease.** GORD is the most common digestive disease. Obesity and alcohol excess are two significant risk factors for this condition. Heartburn and acid reflux are common presentations of GORD; extra-oesophageal acid reflux can also occur with a variety of upper and lower respiratory symptoms as listed in Chapter 5. Although GORD is a clinical diagnosis, urgent upper GI endoscopy should be considered in any patients with 'red flag' symptoms and/or early-onset persistent dyspepsia in those over 55 (see MICRO-facts box in Chapter 5).

Barrett's oesophagus is a combined histological and endoscopic diagnosis, which cannot be diagnosed from symptoms alone. Achalasia tends to present with dysphagia, chest pain, regurgitation and weight loss, none of which were present in the history. Candidiasis and eosinophilic oesophagitis usually cause dysphagia and odynophagia. Gastric volvulus causes epigastric pain, retching without vomiting or early post-prandial vomiting. There are no alarm symptoms suggestive of oesophageal cancer. Although pharyngeal pouch can cause chronic cough, it is usually associated with dysphagia and regurgitation. Adult patients with tracheal-oesophageal fistula usually have previous history of malignancy or radiotherapy; clinical presentation is with an intermittent choking feeling, dysphagia and recurrent lower respiratory tract infection.

Answer 18

1) **Achalasia.** This condition is a neuropathic motor disorder of the oesophageal smooth muscle. Common presenting symptoms are dysphagia to both solids and liquids, regurgitation and weight loss. Barium swallow is a helpful test in showing oesophageal dilatation, while typical manometry findings show low amplitude, non-propagating contractions with failure of the lower oesophageal sphincter to relax on swallowing. Normal OGD and oesophageal biopsies should exclude the conditions above apart from gastric volvulus, which causes acute symptoms of abdominal pain and vomiting, and gastro-oesophageal reflux in which two-thirds of patients can have normal endoscopic findings, but weight loss is not typical of this condition in the absence of complications.

Answer 19

8) **Oesophageal cancer.** This patient reports two red flag symptoms suggestive of oesophageal cancer (weight loss and dysphagia). Considering his age and background history of Barrett's oesophagus, oesophageal cancer should be first in the list of differential diagnoses. Although other conditions like eosinophilic oesophagitis and achalasia can also cause dysphagia and weight loss, the fairly rapid sequence of events in a patient of this age makes oesophageal malignancy the most likely diagnosis.

OESOPHAGUS: SBA

Answer 20

1) **All of the options.** PPI therapy alongside lifestyle modification should all be considered in this otherwise fit and healthy patient with no red flag symptoms.

Answer 21

5) **Oesophageal spasm.** Barium swallow findings are very suggestive of oesophageal spasm. A normal gastroscopy and oesophageal biopsies exclude Barrett's oesophagus and eosinophilic oesophagitis. Dysphagia is uncommon in uncomplicated oesophagitis and if it occurs, it is usually to solids. Achalasia is possible but is usually associated with reduced peristalsis and hold-up at the gastro-oesophageal junction.

STOMACH AND DUODENUM: EMQ

Answer 22

2) **Domperidone.** This patient is suffering from gastroparesis. Domperidone stimulates peristalsis causing relief of symptoms. The diagnosis can usually be confirmed by radiolabelled scintigraphy or electrophysiological tests.

Self-assessment

Further surgical intervention or possibly a gastric pacemaker may be considered if pharmacological intervention is unsuccessful in controlling the symptoms.

Answer 23

3) **Endoscopic haemostatic therapy.** The man probably has a peptic ulcer that has eroded through a blood vessel causing haemorrhage (remember, posterior ulcers pose an increased risk of haemorrhage due to proximity to the gastroduodenal artery). He has had a recent myocardial infarction and is likely to be on antiplatelet therapy. Endoscopy with a view to haemostatic therapy is the initial treatment option of choice for suspected bleeding peptic ulcers. A PPI should be started after the gastroscopy has determined the cause of the bleeding and given intravenously if the ulcer is thought to be at high risk of rebleeding.

Answer 24

4) **Endoscopic mucosal resection.** EMR is the treatment of choice for gastric carcinoma that is confined to the mucosa. This involves injecting fluid into the submucosal layer to lift the tumour away from the underlying muscularis propria and then removing this with an electrical snare. A similar technique known as endoscopic submucosal dissection (ESD), which, following injection of fluid into the submucosal layers uses an electrical cutting knife through the endoscope to cut beneath the tumour to allow this to be removed in a single piece, is also used but is not so widely available in the UK. For more advanced carcinoma without local or regional spread, gastrectomy may be considered alongside chemotherapy.

STOMACH AND DUODENUM: SBA

Answer 25

2) **Schilling test.** Initial tests for pernicious anaemia would include FBC, serum vitamin B_{12} and autoantibodies. The Schilling test provides a confirmatory diagnosis as it differentiates pernicious anaemia from other megaloblastic anaemias. Approximately 80–85% of patients with pernicious anaemia have positive anti-gastric parietal cell antibodies and 50% have positive anti-intrinsic factor antibodies.

Answer 26

1) **Adenocarcinoma.** Adenocarcinoma accounts for 90% of gastric cancers with the remaining 10% being made up of lymphomas (5%), carcinoid tumours, GISTs and other rare tumours.

Answer 27

4) **Pyloric stenting.** This woman has an advanced gastric cancer with liver metastases. With her poor exercise tolerance, surgery would likely carry a high risk of anaesthetic complications. Endoscopic stenting is a minimally invasive procedure that will relieve the outlet obstruction and would pose much less of a risk for this particular patient. Gastric tumours rarely respond well to radiotherapy, so this intervention is not indicated here.

THE SMALL BOWEL: EMQs

EMQ 1

Answer 28

2) **Coeliac disease.** This patient has steatorrhoea, characteristic of malabsorption. Her increasing fatigue is probably related to her anaemia and low iron and folic acid levels due to malabsorption as a result of her coeliac disease. While the classic coeliac disease patient is a young child with poor growth, many patients now present later in life with a long history of non-specific GI symptoms. Whipple's disease can present in a similar way but is more common in males and is much less prevalent than coeliac disease (1% of the population have coeliac disease). Lactose intolerance can also cause diarrhoea but it is unlikely to cause steatorrhoea. Small intestinal bacterial overgrowth is more common in diabetics and can cause steatorrhoea, but usually causes B_{12} deficiency rather than iron and folic acid deficiency. The long symptom history suggests an infective cause is unlikely.

Answer 29

6) **Small bowel carcinoid tumour.** The symptoms displayed here are suggestive of carcinoid syndrome. The release of serotonin and other vasoactive substances from a carcinoid tumour causes a range of symptoms including facial flushing, diarrhoea, vomiting and dyspnoea. Other than vomiting, this patient is demonstrating all of these symptoms. The progressive nature is suggestive of a tumour. While other small bowel tumours are listed, they are not associated with the symptoms displayed by this patient.

Answer 30

3) **Lactose intolerance.** Flatulence, bloating, diarrhoea and borborygmi (loud rumbling of the stomach) are associated with lactose intolerance. Lactose reaching the small bowel is metabolized by colonic bacteria with resultant release of large amounts of gas. The increased osmotic gradient draws water into the colon causing the diarrhoea. Lactose intolerance is far more common in particular populations, particularly patients from an Asian background.

Whipple's disease and coeliac disease also present with similar abdominal symptoms. Whipple's disease is mainly found in white, middle-aged males, while coeliac disease is less common in Asian populations.

EMQ 2

Answer 31

7) ***Staphylococcus aureus.*** The rapid onset of symptoms after exposure suggests this is a toxin-mediated form of gastroenteritis. These infections have a rapid onset of symptoms as they are caused by the ingestion of pre-formed toxins and therefore do not require time for multiplication of pathogens. Other than *Bacillus cereus*, which is also toxin mediated, all the other infections listed have a longer incubation time. *Staph. aureus* infection is commonly contracted from contaminated foods such as those served at this children's party and has a short duration of around 24 hours. *Bacillus cereus* infection is commonly contracted from fried rice and so is unlikely following a child's party.

Answer 32

2) ***Campylobacter* spp.** This infection commonly causes profuse diarrhoea that can be bloody in some patients and has a duration of 5–7 days. It is commonly contracted from undercooked poultry, contaminated water and milk. It is associated with Guillain–Barré syndrome, a post-infective demyelinating neuropathy that causes ascending weakness.

Answer 33

3) ***Clostridium difficile.*** *Clostridium difficile* infection is common following a course of antibiotics, which this patient had for a recent UTI, especially in the elderly. Antibiotics disrupt the normal flora of the GI tract allowing *C. difficile*, a common bacterium which naturally resides in the intestine of many humans, to proliferate. Overgrowth can cause a pseudomembranous colitis with inflammation and disruption of the normal function of the colon. While the other bacteria listed can cause diarrhoea, this case is a classic *C. difficile* presentation.

THE SMALL BOWEL: SBA

Answer 34

1) **Cholecystokinin.** CCK is one of two hormones listed that is secreted in response to amino acids in the small intestine – the other is somatostatin. While CCK stimulates pancreatic enzyme secretion and gallbladder contraction, somatostatin is a largely inhibitory hormone which decreases gallbladder motility. Gastrin is secreted in response to stimuli in the stomach. The final two hormones are released in response to small bowel stimuli but not amino acids.

Answer 35

5) **Tissue transglutaminase.** tTG is the first-line immunological investigation in suspected coeliac disease. EMA is used if tTG is unavailable or the result is equivocal as it is less sensitive but more specific. Both EMA and tTG are IgA antibodies and since there is an increased incidence of IgA deficiency in patients with coeliac disease, this test should be performed along with a measurement of IgA levels. IgA deficiency is not specific in coeliac disease and is only deficient in 2.6% of cases and is therefore not a good screening test alone. IELs are intra-epithelial lymphocytes, a common finding on duodenal biopsy in coeliac disease patients. HLA is the tissue type. Two tissue types are associated with coeliac disease, HLA DQ2 and DQ8.

Answer 36

4) **Small intestinal bacterial overgrowth.** While most of the conditions listed can present with similar symptoms, a positive hydrogen breath test is associated with small intestinal bacterial overdose and lactose intolerance. In small bowel bacterial overdose, the hydrogen is released as bacteria in the small bowel metabolize orally ingested lactulose or glucose. In lactose intolerance, hydrogen is released following ingestion of lactose from metabolism of the non-absorbed lactose within the large intestine. The macrocytosis suggests malabsorption of B_{12} or folic acid. B_{12} deficiency is common in bacterial overgrowth and is not seen in lactose intolerance. Coeliac disease can cause a macrocytosis, usually due to folic acid deficiency (occasionally due to B_{12} deficiency), and can also be associated with lactose intolerance. However the negative anti-tTG makes the diagnosis unlikely. Small bowel lymphoma is associated with coeliac disease but doesn't tend to present in this way.

COLORECTAL DISEASE: EMQs

EMQ 1

Answer 37

1) **Acute diverticulitis.** 80% of people aged 85 and older in Western countries have diverticular disease. About 20% of those will develop acute diverticulitis. The typical presentation of acute diverticulitis includes abdominal pain, rectal bleeding, fever, nausea and altered bowel habit. Although inflammatory bowel disease could be a possibility, it usually has a more subacute course at presentation. Acute colitis usually presents with a gradual worsening of symptoms over several days to weeks. Small bowel obstruction does not cause rectal bleeding unless it is complicated by bowel ischaemia/infarction. Similarly, coeliac disease, irritable bowel syndrome and prostatitis do not cause rectal bleeding.

Answer 38

6) **Inflammatory bowel disease.** Common symptoms of Crohn's disease activity include weight loss and abdominal pain with or without diarrhoea. The inflammatory markers are usually elevated, more markedly in extensive, severe disease (raised platelets, CRP, ESR, WCC and ferritin). Significant weight loss is not consistent with irritable bowel syndrome or chronic constipation. Negative coeliac serology makes coeliac disease very unlikely. The subacute nature of presentation in this scenario makes diagnosis of small bowel obstruction or acute diverticulitis unlikely. Uncomplicated benign ovarian cyst does not cause general malaise, weight loss or raised inflammatory markers.

Answer 39

7) **Irritable bowel syndrome–constipation predominant (IBS-C).** The symptoms suggest IBS with predominant constipation; lack of red flag symptoms and normal screening blood tests exclude the inflammatory processes listed above. The absence of nocturnal symptoms makes other diagnoses less likely. As the patient has associated abdominal pain and bloating, the diagnosis is not chronic constipation. Benign ovarian cyst can present with chronic pelvic pain but the rest of the symptoms are not supportive of this diagnosis. Chronicity of the symptoms is not supportive of acute bowel obstruction or diverticulitis.

EMQ 2

Answer 40

5) **IV hydrocortisone.** The patient's symptoms and laboratory test results indicate severe acute ulcerative colitis as per the Truelove criteria (see MICRO-facts box in Chapter 8). The patient should therefore be treated with IV hydrocortisone alongside prophylactic low molecular weight heparin. IV ciclosporin or infliximab is considered as the second-line medical therapy if the patient does not respond to IV hydrocortisone by day 3. Emergency colectomy would be an alternative to medical therapy if the patient fails to respond or if the patient's condition further deteriorates at any point. Thiopurines, methotrexate and budesonide are not suitable for treatment of acute severe ulcerative colitis.

Answer 41

10) **Thiopurines.** Azathioprine or 6-mercaptopurine (thiopurines) should be considered as first-line maintenance therapy in Crohn's disease following an acute severe attack or if two (or more) relapses requiring steroids occur in a 12-month period. Methotrexate is generally the second-line maintenance therapy in patients intolerant to thiopurines. Infliximab can also be used as a third-line option for maintenance therapy in Crohn's disease. Corticosteroids should not be used as the long-term maintenance therapy option.

Answer 42

9) **Prucalopride.** Following current NICE guidelines, prucalopride should be considered in women with chronic constipation who have not responded to at least two laxatives from different classes at the highest tolerated dose for at least 6 months. Increasing oral fluid intake together with regular exercise and a high-fibre diet are generally the first-line non-pharmacological approaches for the treatment of chronic constipation. Surgical intervention is the last resort in the line of chronic constipation management.

COLORECTAL DISEASE: SBAs

SBA 1

Answer 43

2) **CEA.** This test should not be conducted as part of a screening for IBS. It should only be used for monitoring recurrence in patients with previous colorectal cancer (see Section 8.10).

SBA 2

Answer 44

4) **Ischaemic colitis.** This patient's symptoms and background medical history are suggestive of ischaemic colitis. AXR findings are supportive of the diagnosis and exclude acute bowel obstruction. Elevated serum lactate also raises the suspicion of bowel ischaemia. Although colorectal cancer is always a feasible diagnosis in an elderly patient with rectal bleeding, the acute presentation of this scenario makes this diagnosis a less likely option. Abdominal pain, rectal bleeding and raised WCC could be a sign of acute diverticulitis but not chronic diverticular disease. Melanosis coli is a benign disorder manifested as brown hyperpigmentation of the colonic mucosa usually secondary to chronic laxative overuse.

PANCREATOBILIARY DISEASE: EMQ

Answer 45

7) **Laparoscopic cholecystectomy.** This woman is suffering from gallstones. The gold standard management for symptomatic gallstones is surgical removal of the gallbladder. Dissolution therapy and shock wave lithotripsy are rarely used in patients who are fit for surgery.

Answer 46

6) **IV fluids.** This man has a case of acute pancreatitis, likely to be caused by alcoholism. Although ERCP may be required later if gallstones are suspected as

the cause, supportive treatment for pancreatitis includes immediate administration of IV 0.9% saline.

Answer 47

8) **Pancreaticoduodenectomy.** This patient's pancreatic carcinoma shows a good chance of complete resection, and although adjuvant chemotherapy may be considered, a Whipple's procedure is the definitive treatment.

PANCREATOBILIARY DISEASE: SBA

Answer 48

5) **Trousseau's sign (thrombophlebitis migrans).** Thrombophlebitis migrans affects multiple vessels within the limbs at different times and is associated with a thrombotic state that should make the clinician suspicious of malignancy (most commonly associated with lung or pancreatic carcinoma). Both Cullen's and Grey Turner's signs are associated with pancreatitis. Murphy's sign is indicative of gallstones and Courvoisier's sign may indicate gallbladder carcinoma.

Answer 49

1) **Adenocarcinoma.** Although small cell carcinoma, squamous cell carcinoma, sarcoma and neuroendocrine tumours are all histological subtypes of gallbladder cancer, adenocarcinoma is the most common presentation.

Answer 50

5) **Proteolytic enzymes.** The pancreas secretes all of the above substances; however, only proteolytic enzymes are stored in their inactive form to prevent autodigestion of pancreatic tissue.

LIVER DISEASE: EMQs

EMQ 1

Answer 51

9) **Primary sclerosing cholangitis.** This patient is showing typical presenting features and risk associated with PSC. A diagnosis of viral hepatitis or alcohol-related liver disease is unlikely, as the patient has no history of past risk-taking behaviours (IV drug use, consumption of contaminated foods, excessive alcohol consumption etc.). Although other autoimmune conditions such as PBC and autoimmune hepatitis should be considered, the fact that the patient is P-ANCA positive means that a diagnosis of PSC is more likely.

Answer 52

6) **Hepatitis E.** The patient is clearly exhibiting several of the clinical features associated with hepatitis. The patient's age combined with the fact that she is feverish suggests a viral rather than an autoimmune mechanism. Since she has confessed to eating local cuisine and has possibly been staying in areas of poor sanitation, hepatitis A or E appears to be the most likely diagnosis, as both are transmitted by the faecal–oral route. She has been inoculated against hepatitis A which is effective in approximately 90% of cases, so this makes hepatitis A unlikely.

Answer 53

2) **Autoimmune hepatitis.** This patient is showing typical symptoms of hepatitis. Her lack of risk factors (poor sanitation, IV drug use, excessive alcohol consumption etc.) makes a diagnosis of viral hepatitis or alcohol-induced liver disease less likely. In this case, the patient's arthralgia may be explained as an extrahepatic feature of autoimmune hepatitis; autoimmune hepatitis is also strongly associated with an ANA-positive status.

EMQ 2

Answer 54

3) **Hepatitis B.** This man is from sub-Saharan Africa. The incidence of hepatitis B is high in this area. It is likely the man contracted hepatitis B many years ago, causing slow and gradual cirrhosis of the liver predisposing him to HCC. The prevalence of hepatitis B and HCC is very closely linked. It is possible the HCC was caused by another source of cirrhosis. Hepatitis C is possible although less common than hepatitis B. If the patient had a history of alcohol misuse ALD may be the cause, likewise if the patient was obese then cirrhosis may have resulted from NAFLD. Hereditary haemochromatosis and Wilson's disease can cause cirrhosis but are both uncommon.

Answer 55

7) **Metastatic liver disease.** 90% of liver masses are metastatic in origin. HCC is uncommon and associated with previous liver disease. Although the other illnesses can cause jaundice and liver failure, multiple masses suggest a malignancy.

Answer 56

6) **Hereditary haemochromatosis.** Erectile dysfunction results from iron deposition in the pituitary and gonads. Polydipsia is a sign of diabetes mellitus secondary to pancreatic damage due to iron deposition and the knee pain is likely due to chondrocalcinosis. All of these features are associated with

haemochromatosis. Wilson's disease can cause neurological and psychiatric problems but is less common than haemochromatosis. The familial aspect of this presentation makes the other illnesses less likely.

LIVER DISEASE: SBA

Answer 57

4) **Hepatitis B surface antibody.** Hepatitis B surface antibody found in isolation usually indicates that the patient has acquired immunity following vaccination. The presence of hepatitis B antigens in the serology generally suggests that the patient is actively suffering from viral hepatitis or has previously contracted the disease. Hepatitis B envelope antibody suggests loss of hepatitis B envelope antigen and a reduction in viral load and infectivity. However such patients still have hepatitis B surface antigen and hence are still infected with the hepatitis B virus until this is also lost with the development of hepatitis B surface antibodies.

Answer 58

1) **Cholestyramine.** Cholestyramine is used as a first-line medication in the treatment of pruritis. Ursodeoxycholic acid is used to slow disease progression in PBC but is not used to directly treat pruritis. Pegylated interferon-α is used in the management of viral hepatitis.

Answer 59

1) **Alcoholic liver disease.** Although this finding is associated with NAFLD, Wilson's disease and HCC, it is most commonly found in biopsy specimens from patients with alcohol-related liver disease.

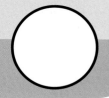

Index